# Contents

# Animal Biology and Care

**S. E. Dallas**
*VN, CertEd*

**b**

**Blackwell
Science**

© 2000 by
Blackwell Science Ltd
Editorial Offices:
Osney Mead, Oxford OX2 0EL
25 John Street, London WC1N 2BL
23 Ainslie Place, Edinburgh EH3 6AJ
350 Main Street, Malden
  MA 02148 5018, USA
54 University Street, Carlton
  Victoria 3053, Australia
10, rue Casimir Delavigne
  75006 Paris, France

Other Editorial Offices:

Blackwell Wissenschafts-Verlag GmbH
Kurfürstendamm 57
10707 Berlin, Germany

Blackwell Science KK
MG Kodenmacho Building
7–10 Kodenmacho Nihombashi
Chuo-ku, Tokyo 104, Japan

First published 2000

Set in 10/13 pt Times
by Best-set Typesetter Ltd., Hong Kong
Printed and bound in Great Britain by
MPG Books, Bodmin, Cornwall

The Blackwell Science logo is a
trade mark of Blackwell Science Ltd,
registered at the United Kingdom
Trade Marks Registry

DISTRIBUTORS
Marston Book Services Ltd
PO Box 269
Abingdon
Oxon OX14 4YN
(*Orders*: Tel: 01235 465500
         Fax: 01235 465555)

USA
Blackwell Science, Inc.
Commerce Place
350 Main Street
Malden, MA 02148 5018
(*Orders*: Tel: 800 759 6102
                781 388 8250
         Fax: 781 388 8255)

Canada
Login Brothers Book Company
324 Saulteaux Crescent
Winnipeg, Manitoba R3J 3T2
(*Orders*: Tel: 204 837 2987
         Fax: 204 837 3116)

Australia
Blackwell Science Pty Ltd
54 University Street
Carlton, Victoria 3053
(*Orders*: Tel: 03 9347 0300
         Fax: 03 9347 5001)

A catalogue record for this title
is available from the British Library

ISBN 0-632-05054-3

Library of Congress
Cataloging-in-Publication Data
Dallas, Sue.
    Animal biology and care/Sue Dallas.
    p.  cm.
    Includes bibliographical references and index.
    ISBN 0-632-05054-3 (pbk.)
    1. Veterinary medicine.  I. Title.
SF745.D246  2000
636.089′073–dc21                    99-38885
                                    CIP

For further information on
Blackwell Science, visit our website:
www.blackwell-science.com

# Preface

The motivation for this book was to provide information necessary to the initial Animal Care and Veterinary Nurse (Pre-Veterinary Nurse) courses in one place. As such, this book is intended as a foundation text for both subjects. I hope the reader will find it a useful and enjoyable introduction.

This book grew from the need, in the animal care sector particularly, for texts to help in training and examinations. My hope is that it will also appeal to a wider audience of animal carers. With a better understanding and knowledge of the care required by animals, in particular mammals, injury and ill health can be better managed. The basic principles of nursing remain unchanged whether carried out at home or within a veterinary practice hospital. Methods for the control or elimination of disease are the same whether one is dealing with a single animal or a large group, for example in a kennel, cattery or animal collection.

The book format seeks to provide information in a readily accessible layout and the text is illustrated with line drawings and photographs. It is divided into three sections, each concentrating on a specific area.

- Section 1 – Animal science. This introduces the reader to basic cell and tissue structure through to organ structures and systems. Both the anatomy and physiology (function) of the organs and organ systems are covered.
- Section 2 – Animal health and husbandry. This takes the reader through the basic requirements for animal health, concentrating on disease transfer and the effect of micro-organisms on body systems.
- Section 3 – Nursing. This covers the nursing procedures for an animal both before and after professional attention from a veterinary surgeon, with an introduction to medical terminology.

I am grateful to the staff of Blackwell Science for their help, particularly Antonia Seymour for her guidance during the writing process; to family and friends for their support and encouragement throughout; and to past and future students, whose need for a course text led me to write this book.

*Sue Dallas*
*VN, CertEd*

# Section 1
# Animal Biology

# Chapter 1
# Cells and Basic Tissue

## Biology – the study of life and living organisms

### But what is life?

This is best answered by stating what distinguishes a living organism from a non-living organism. In order to be considered alive, the following are essential·

- *Growth* – from within by a process which involves the intake of new materials from the outside and their incorporation in the internal structure of the organism.
- *Movement* – the organism is capable of moving itself or a part of itself.
- *Excretion* – the removal of the waste products of metabolism.
- *Eating* – taking in materials to maintain life and growth.
- *Responsiveness* – to stimuli in its surroundings.
- *Release of energy* – in a controlled and usable form.

> Therefore considering units of life:
>
> *Cells* form . . .
> *Tissues*, and tissues form . . .
> *Organs*, and organs have a . . .
> *Function* to perform in the living organism!

The cell is the functional unit of all tissues and has the ability to perform individually all the essential life functions. Within the various tissues of the body, the constituent cells show a wide range of specialisations. However, all cells conform to a basic model of cell structure.

### The diversity of cells

All cells are not identical (Fig. 1.1) but all have the same basic features:

- Chromosomes
- Mitochondria

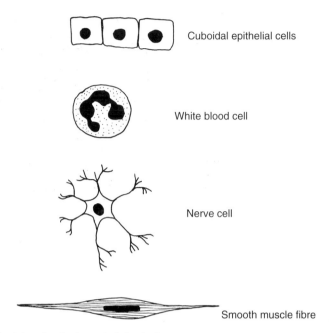

Cuboidal epithelial cells

White blood cell

Nerve cell

Smooth muscle fibre

**Fig. 1.1** Diversity of cells from their basic form.

- Endoplasmic reticulum
- Ribosomes

The above are common to virtually all cells but the shape, form and contents of individual cells show much variation. The structural characteristics of a particular cell are closely related to its functions.

- *Epithelial cells* – have a shape and form that makes them most suitable for lining the surface of the body and the organs and cavities within it.
- *Glandular cells* – are responsible for producing some kind of secretion, for example mucus to lubricate between tissues.
- *Osteoblasts* – produce bone tissue.
- *Erythrocytes* (*red blood cells*) – have a shape designed to hold the red pigment haemoglobin which conveys oxygen around the body. In order to do this, they are one of the few cells in the body which no longer contain a nucleus.
- *Nerve cells* – or neurones, have slender arm-like processes which will transmit electrical impulses through the nervous system to reach the whole body.
- *Muscle cells* – are also capable of electrical activity accompanied by a muscle contraction for body movement.

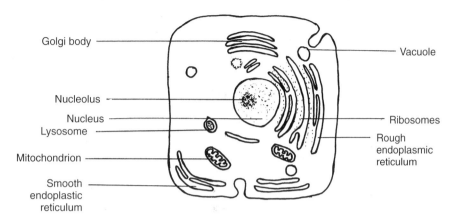

**Fig. 1.2** Basic cell structure.

# Cells

Cells have the same basic structure no matter what their function is or what organism they are found in (Fig. 1.2). Therefore the single cell which forms the body of an amoeba and the brain cell of a dog have certain features in common. All cells contain:

* A *nucleus* – to control the cell's activities
* *Cytoplasm* – a jelly-like material to support organs
* *Cell membrane* – this encloses the cytoplasm in which lies the nucleus

These three parts make up *protoplasm* – living matter.
For life, cells require:

* Food for energy
* Water (body fluid) to hydrate the cells
* Oxygen to all cells
* Suitable temperature in which to live

## The nucleus

At least one nucleus is found in the cells of all organisms. The nucleus of a cell contains rod-shaped objects called *chromosomes*. These are only visible when a cell is about to divide into two. Chromosomes contain a complex chemical called *deoxyribonucleic acid (DNA)*. DNA controls the development of the features that an organism inherits from its parents. In other words, it contains the chemical 'instructions' for making an organism.

### The cell membrane

The cell membrane is 0.00001 mm thick and forms the outer boundary of the cell. It is here that all exchanges take place between a cell and its surrounding environment. In a manner which is not yet fully understood, this membrane allows certain chemicals to pass in and out of the cell but prevents the passage of others (referred to as *osmosis*). As a result, the cell membranes are said to be *selectively permeable*.

### The cytoplasm

The term *cytoplasm* refers to all the living substances of a cell except the nucleus. Cytoplasm is a jelly-like material containing a large number of important substances, many of which are concerned with metabolism.

- *Organelles* – are the structures visible within the cell other than the nucleus.
- *Mitochondria* – are one of the most important organelles, where chemical reactions of respiration take place. This is the release of energy for cellular function.
- *Rough endoplasmic reticulum* – has ribosomes on it that have been produced in the nucleus. Protein is synthesised here and the cell may transport it for use in the manufacture of digestive enzymes and hormones.
- *Smooth endoplasmic reticulum* – does not have ribosomes but is concerned with the synthesis and transport of lipids (fats) and steroids of body origin.
- *Ribosomes* – are granules rich in ribonucleic acid, in which protein is synthesised.
- *Centrosome* – lies near the nucleus and is made up of two *centrioles*. It is important during cell division and the formation of the cilia and flagella of certain cells (the slender projecting hairs for movement of single-celled organisms).
- *Lysosomes* – are dark round bodies containing enzymes responsible for splitting complex chemical compounds into simpler ones (known as *lysis*, meaning 'to break up') followed by digestion. They also destroy worn-out organelles within the cell. These destructive enzymes are stored in tubes in the cell called the *Golgi complex or body*.

## Basic tissue

Tissues are a collection of cells and their products, which have a common fundamental function and in which one particular type of cell predominates.

- *Epithelial* – which forms a protective layer both inside and on the surface of the body. Examples of this tissue are skin, glands and the linings of the various body systems.
- *Connective* – which supports tissues and acts as a transport system to move materials vital to tissue cells around the body. Examples of this tissue are:
  (a)  loose connective tissue which surrounds organs
  (b)  dense connective tissue which has great strength and is found as tendons and ligaments
  (c)  blood which transports essential nutrients, gases, waste products, hormones and enzymes to and from all body cells
  (d)  cartilage and bone which provide shape and protection for organs and allow movement.
- *Muscular* – tissues concerned with movement of the skeleton, organ systems and the heart.
- *Nervous* – which transports messages to tissues, connecting the body as a whole for the required response.

### Epithelial tissue

This tissue covers all surfaces of the body, both inside and out, be it a surface, a cavity or a tube. It is made up of a diverse group of tissues which are involved in a wide range of activities such as secretion of a special fluid, protection and absorption.

Depending on their function, the cells of this tissue will have a varied shape, structure and thickness. They are classified according to appearance:

- *Number of layers* – a single layer of these cells is called *simple epithelium*; more than one layer is called *stratified epithelium*.
- *Shape* of the cells involved.
- *Specialisations*, such as tiny hairs called cilia or special thickened surface tissue called keratin, which covers the nose and pads of the feet.
- *Glandular* – meaning it is involved in secretion. Secretions which go directly into the bloodstream are called *hormones* and are produced by glands of the *endocrine* or *ductless system*. If the gland has a duct it will secrete onto a surface and belongs to the *exocrine system*; for example, enzymes secreted by the pancreas.

The many and varied functions of epithelial tissue mean that it will take different forms. There are six main types.

*Pavement* – found lining surfaces involved in the transport of gases (lungs) or fluids (walls of blood vessels) (Fig. 1.3a).
*Cuboidal* – which lines small ducts and tubes like those of the kidney, pancreas and salivary glands of the mouth (Fig. 1.3b).
*Columnar* – located on highly absorbing surfaces like the small intestine for the uptake of nutrients (Fig. 1.3c).

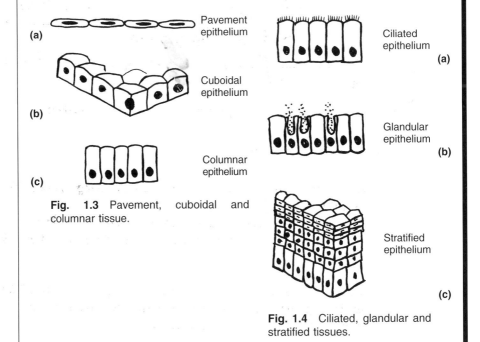

**Fig. 1.3** Pavement, cuboidal and columnar tissue.

**Fig. 1.4** Ciliated, glandular and stratified tissues.

*Ciliated* – has tiny hair-like projections in parallel rows on the surface of the cell, which beat in a wave-like manner, moving films of mucus or fluid in a particular direction. For example, in the respiratory airway (trachea), they remove unwanted inhaled materials (Fig. 1.4a).
*Glandular* – which secrete a special fluid containing hormones or enzymes (Fig. 1.4b).
*Stratified* – this type of epithelium has two or more layers of cells. Its function is mostly protection. Found lining the mouth cavity or as skin (Fig. 1.4c).

### Connective tissue

This tissue binds all the other body tissues together. It supports them and acts as a transport system for the exchange of nutrients, metabolites and waste products between tissues and the circulatory system (Fig. 1.5).

Connective tissues occur in many different forms with a wide range of physical properties.

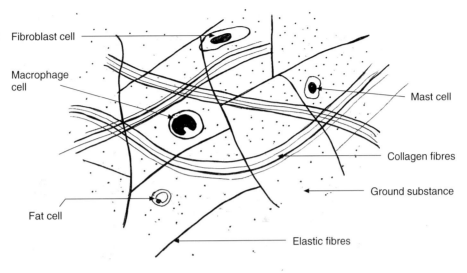

Fibroblast cell

Macrophage cell

Mast cell

Collagen fibres

Ground substance

Fat cell

Elastic fibres

**Fig. 1.5**  Connective tissue.

- *Loose* connective tissue acts as a type of packing material between other tissues with specific functions.
- *Dense* connective tissue provides tough support in the skin.
- *Rigid* forms of connective tissue, like cartilage and bone, support the skeleton.

Connective tissue also has functions including the storage of fat in adipose tissue, fighting infection with micro-organisms and tissue repair.

Connective tissue has two components.

(1)  *Cells*:
- fibroblasts for repair and maintenance of the tissue
- fat-storing cells
- defence and immune function cells called *macrophages.*
(2)  Material called *ground substance* which holds together other materials to make up tissue and looks like a semifluid gel.

Connective tissue is composed of two types of fibre.

- *Collagen* – produced by the fibroblasts, is not elastic but has great tensile strength. Tendons by which muscles are attached to bones are composed of collagen fibres.
- *Elastin* – has great elasticity and is found in ligaments which bind bones of the skeleton together.

Connective tissue can be described as a mixture of fibres in different proportions. Its efficiency in binding structures together is achieved by the special grouping of proteins in the ground substance. The particular type and abundance of fibre present depend on the stresses and strains to which the tissue is normally subjected.

# Blood

This is a highly specialised tissue consisting of several types of cell suspended in a fluid medium called *plasma*. The cellular constituents consist of:

- Red blood cells (erythrocytes)
- White blood cells (leucocytes)
- Platelets (thrombocytes)

Blood has a varied structure and performs a wide range of functions. One of its main functions is that of transportation, of the red blood cells around the body and all the materials in the plasma. Blood is considered a tissue because it connects all the cells in the body together.

Live animals constantly absorb useful substances like oxygen and food, which must then be distributed throughout their bodies. They produce a continuous stream of waste materials, such as carbon dioxide, which must be removed from their bodies before they reach harmful levels. The distribution of food, oxygen and other substances throughout the body and the removal of any wastes is performed by this transport system tissue.

## Composition of the blood

Fluid called *plasma* makes up about 60%. Cells and other material in transit make up the remaining 40%.

If a sample of blood (mixed with an anticoagulant to stop it clotting) was put into a centrifuge and spun to separate out the component parts, it would show at the top of the tube the fluid part (plasma), then the platelets (cell fragments), then the white blood cells and finally the red cells (Fig. 1.6).

### Plasma

This is mainly water containing a variety of dissolved substances which are transported from one part of the body to another. To give a few examples, food materials (glucose, lipids and amino acids) are conveyed from the small intestine to the liver; urea from the liver to the kidneys; hormones from various ductless glands to their target organs. Cells are constantly shedding materials into the blood which flows past them and removing materials from it. Plasma provides the medium through which this continual exchange takes place.

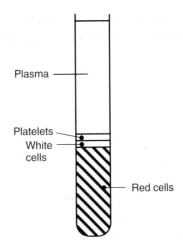

**Fig. 1.6**  Blood separated into layers.

| PLASMA | SERUM |
|---|---|
| FIBRINOGEN (protein for clotting) **plus** water, protein, glucose, lipids, amino acids, salts, enzymes, hormones and waste products | Contains water, protein, glucose, lipids, amino acids, salts, enzymes, hormones and waste products **but** no proteins for clotting (these have been used up) |

Plasma carries many more products than the diagram shows, including the plasma proteins called albumin, globulin and fibrinogen. Fibrinogen plays an important role in the process of blood clotting. When it has been used up by clot formation then the fluid part of blood seen at the site of injury is called *serum*. Therefore, serum is plasma with the fibrinogen removed. About 92% of blood is made of water and this same water can be forced into the tissues. It is then called *tissue fluid* because of its location.

It is important to realise that plasma and the tissue fluid derived from it form the environment which keeps body cells alive. In a sense, these fluids are equivalent to a pond or fish tank in which both single-celled organisms and multicelled organisms live and are supplied with their food and oxygen and into which they excrete waste.

### Red blood cells (erythrocytes)

These are produced in the red or active bone marrow. The main function of red blood cells is to carry oxygen from the respiratory organ to the tissues and their structure is modified accordingly. These cells have had their nucleus removed, with the result that the cell is sunk in on each side, giving it the shape of a biconcave disc. It is surrounded by a thin elastic membrane and the interior of the cell

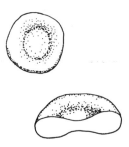

**Fig. 1.7**  Cross-section of a red blood cell showing its biconcave shape.

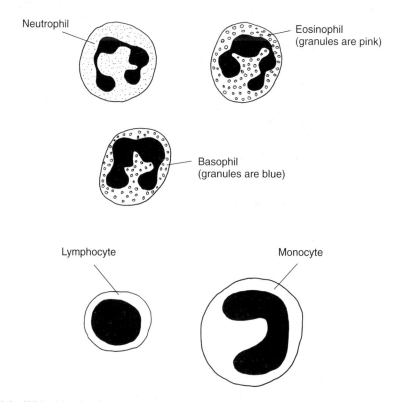

**Fig. 1.8**  White blood cells.

is filled with the red pigment haemoglobin which combines with and carries oxygen (Fig. 1.7).

### White blood cells (leucocytes)

The white cells are fewer in number and have a very different role to play. They fall into two groups (Fig. 1.8).

*Granulocytes (granules in the cytoplasm).* These are produced in the bone marrow.

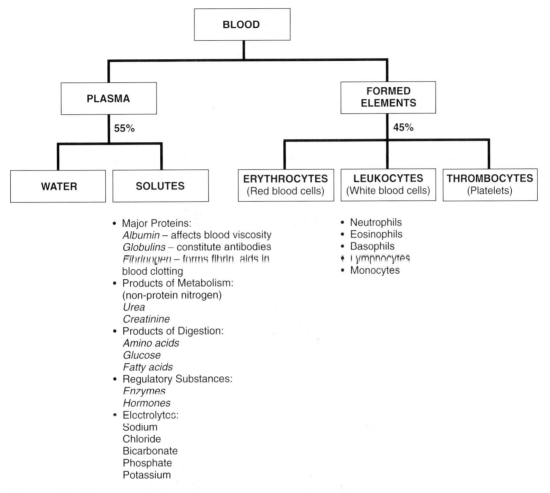

**Fig. 1.9**  Blood components.

- *Neutrophils* – phagocytic cells
- *Eosinophils* – respond to allergies
- *Basophils* – promote inflammation for healing of tissue

*Agranulocytes (no granules in their cytoplasm).*  Produced in the bone marrow or lymph system.

- *Lymphocytes* – support the immune system
- *Monocytes* – phagocyte cells

*Phagocyte* or *phagocytic* means 'cell eater'. These cells eat or engulf other cells / materials that may be harmful and destroy them. Red cells will remain in the bloodstream to perform their role of oxygen carrier but white cells will only use the bloodstream as a transporter from their site of origin to the capillaries where they will push through the wall of the blood vessel and into the tissue spaces. Those that are phagocytic will gather in and around wounds and destroy bacteria and any other harmful material. In this manner the cells assist in 'fighting infection'.

## Bone and cartilage

There are two kinds of skeletal tissue, bone and cartilage.

### Bone

This tissue is closely related to connective tissue, in that it consists of cells embedded in an organic matrix (ground substance). However, this matrix is comparatively hard. The cells of bone are called *osteoblasts* and *osteoclasts*.

### Cartilage

This is a dense, clear, blue/white material which provides support for the body and can be elastic or rigid. Found mainly in joints, it has no blood vessels but is covered by a membrane called the *perichondrium* from which it receives its blood supply. The cells of cartilage are called *chondroblasts*.

There are three types of cartilage:

- *Hyaline* – the cells for hyaline production are called *chondrocytes*. They lie within a hyaline matrix with collagen fibres running through. Hyaline is a smooth tissue and forms articular joint surfaces for bones and the C-shaped rings of cartilage that keep the trachea open for air passage into the lungs.
- *Fibrocartilage* – this is stronger than hyaline but with a similar base structure that contains more collagen fibres. It surrounds the articular surface of some bones, for example in the hip joint (acetabulum) and the shoulder joint (glenoid cavity), and is also found in the stifle or knee joint as pads of cartilage called *menisci*.
- *Elastic* – this has a hyaline matrix and many elastic fibres which provide its elastic properties. It is found in the ear flap (pinna) and in the larynx area of the throat.

## Muscular tissue

The ability to contract is very well developed in this type of tissue. Muscle cells are usually long, thin and thread-like and are often called *fibres*. There are three main types of fibres:

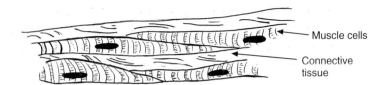

**Fig. 1.10**   Skeletal (striated) muscle fibre.

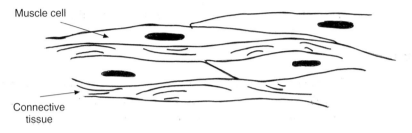

**Fig. 1.11**   Smooth (non-striated) muscle fibre.

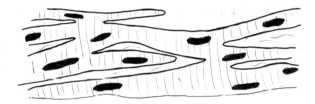

**Fig. 1.12**   Cardiac muscle fibre.

- *Skeletal* (also called voluntary and striated) (Fig. 1.10)
- *Smooth* (also called involuntary, non-striated and visceral) (Fig. 1.11)
- *Cardiac* (Fig. 1.12)

### Skeletal muscle

Found in muscles attached to the skeleton. The cells are cylindrical and vary from about 1 mm to 5 cm in length. Since skeletal muscles respond to the will of the animal, the cells are also called *voluntary* muscle cells.

Skeletal muscles are formed of parallel muscle cells (*fibres*) held together in small bundles by connective tissue. These are collected into larger groups which are also enclosed in connective tissue and ultimately form the muscle which is surrounded by yet more connective tissue commonly called the *muscle sheath*.

When muscles are close to one another, the sheaths may thicken to form an *intermuscular septa*.

All the connective tissue within and around the muscles continues into the connective tissue of the structure to which the muscle is attached, i.e. bone.

Sometimes the muscle appears to attach directly but usually the connective tissue leaves the muscle as a fibrous band known as a *tendon* (i.e. Achilles tendon on the point of the hock) or as a fibrous sheet called an *aponeurosis* (i.e. the sheet of muscle and connective tissue called the diaphragm).

Some muscles are named according to their shape, some according to their functions and others according to their position in the body.

Under the microscope, skeletal muscle cells look striped (they have *striations*).

### Smooth muscle

In direct contrast to skeletal muscle, which is specialised for relatively forceful contractions of short duration and under voluntary control, smooth muscle is specialised for continuous contractions of little force but over a greater section of muscle tissue. For example, the smooth muscle of the intestinal wall contracts in continuous rhythm, moving food through the tract by *peristaltic action*.

These fibres are spindle shaped and about 0.5 mm in length or shorter. Under the microscope they look smooth. Only small amounts of connective tissue bind them together to form sheets or layers of muscle tissue. They may also be called *involuntary* muscles because they are not controlled by the will of the animal. These fibres are found in the muscle of organs, hence the alternative name of *visceral* muscle.

### Cardiac muscle

This muscle produces strong contractions using a lot of energy and is only found in the heart. The contractions are continuous. In order for this to take place, the fibres have junctions or connections with surrounding fibres which allow very rapid contractions of all nearby tissue. The cells are elongated and are the only muscle cells which frequently branch. They are held together by only very small amounts of connective tissue.

## Nervous tissue

The function of this tissue is to transmit electrical messages from one part of the body to another. As a result of this, the nerve cells are interconnected in a very complex way. The cells can transmit and sometimes store information because of this complex link-up with each other.

The cells are called *neurones* (Fig. 1.13) and they connect and communicate to form pathways so that the body can respond to information received. Neurones vary in size and shape depending on where they are in the nervous system. However, all neurones have the same basic structure. They consist of a large cell body containing the nucleus surrounded by cytoplasm, with two types of processes extending from the cell body: a single axon and one or more dendrites.

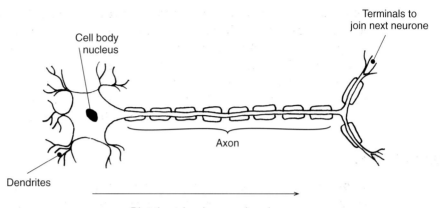

**Fig. 1.13**   A neurone.

*Dendrites* are branched, tapering processes which either end in specialised *sense receptors* (information) or form junctions (*synapses*) with neighbouring neurones from which they receive electrical stimuli, which is passed to the cells beyond.

*Axons* extend from the cell body as a tube-like structure of variable length, carrying stimuli or messages away to the next nerve cell.

# Chapter 2
# Movement of Materials Within the Body

Time now to look at the processes by which materials get into and out of cells. Exchanges can be examined under the following headings:

(1)  Diffusion
(2)  Osmosis
(3)  Phagocytosis
(4)  Active transport

## Diffusion

This is the process of movement of molecules from a region where they are at a comparatively high concentration to a region where they are at a lower concentration, requiring no energy in its achievement. Diffusion will always continue until eventually the molecules are uniformly distributed throughout the system. This is very important in the movement of molecules and salts (electrolytes or ions) in and out of cells.

An example of this process is the cell's requirement for oxygen. It is continually being used up in respiration so the concentration of oxygen inside the cell will be lower than it is in the blood and tissue fluids as a result. Oxygen molecules will diffuse into the cell from outside. With carbon dioxide, the reverse is true: its concentration is highest inside the cells, where it is continually being formed. This results in carbon dioxide molecules diffusing out of the cells.

Anything that increases the concentration of a substance in the body will favour diffusion. Blood is involved here to carry away the diffused substance, so encouraging further diffusion.

## Osmosis

This refers to the movement of water through a semipermeable membrane while expending no energy (Fig. 2.1).

Although the cell wall membrane is fully permeable to respiratory gases, it is not permeable to all substances. The nature of the membrane means that only molecules that are small enough will diffuse through it unimpeded. Larger molecules either penetrate slowly or not at all. The membrane is therefore called *semipermeable*, permitting the passage of some substances but not others.

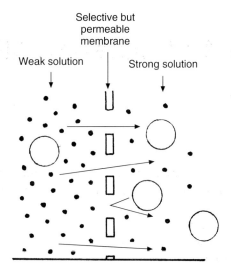

Selective but
permeable
membrane

Weak solution          Strong solution

Large molecules cannot pass through the membrane, but water passes through easily

**Fig. 2.1**   Osmosis.

Osmosis is really a special case of diffusion: it involves the passage of water molecules from a region of high concentration to a region of lower concentration. The concentration will be supplied by other products like salts.

---

**Terms**

*Osmosis* – is the diffusion of fluid through a selectively permeable membrane, from where water is in a high concentration (a *weak solution*) to where water is in a low concentration (a *strong solution*). Osmotic pressure helps to keep fluid in its correct compartment within the body.

*Isotonic* – refers to solutions which cause no transfer of fluid either into or out of a cell. These are the solutions most frequently used in fluid replacement in sick animals, such as 0.9% sodium chloride.

*Hypertonic* – these are solutions with an osmotic pressure higher than that of body fluids. If the cell is surrounded by a solution with an osmotic pressure higher than that of the cell, water passes out of the cell, causing it to shrink.

*Hypotonic* – these are solutions with an osmotic pressure lower than body fluid. In this case the cell is surrounded by almost pure water which allows water to enter cells by osmosis, causing the cell to swell and even to burst.

---

## *Phagocytosis*

The previous headings have outlined how individual molecules cross the cell membrane; this heading covers the larger particles which also need to enter cells. This is achieved by specialised cells which are able to 'cell eat' or *phagocytose*. This process was mentioned when discussing white blood cells which take up and destroy bacteria and other particles which could be harmful to the body.

To phagocytose, the cell membrane changes shape to form a flask-like depression enclosing the particles. The neck of the depression then closes and seals itself off as a food vacuole and migrates towards the centre of the cell. The material is digested by enzymes within the cell. Any useful food products resulting from this process are absorbed into the cell cytoplasm. Phagocytosis is a selective process with the cell distinguishing between food particles and harmful materials.

### Active transport

Diffusion is a purely physical process in which molecules or salts move from a region of higher to a region of lower concentration. But there are certain biological situations where the reverse happens: molecules or salts move from a region of low concentration to a region of higher concentration. They move against the *concentration gradient*. This *active transport* will only take place in a living system that is actively producing energy by respiration. It is not merely a passive barrier but a very active interface between the cell's contents and its immediate surroundings, requiring energy expenditure.

## Body fluid

Dissolved in the body fluids are the essential salts called *electrolytes* or *ions*. They are called electrolytes because they carry one or more electrical charges. Those that are positively charged are called *cations*, i.e. sodium and potassium. Those that are negatively charged are called *anions*, i.e. chloride and bicarbonate.
Their role is to:

* Help control the osmotic pressure
* Assist the pH and buffer mechanisms
* Support the enzyme systems

About 60% of the body consists of fluids. It is divided into two areas:

* Intracellular – 40%
* Extracellular – 20%

Extracellular fluid is further divided into:

* *Tissue fluid* (interstitial) which bathes the tissues and cells
* *Plasma*, which is the water part of blood, needed to transport the cells, nutrients, gases, hormones and waste products

### Acids and bases in the body

The acidity of a solution is expressed as its **pH** (per hydrogen). A pH of 7.0 represents neutral. A solution with a pH of less than 7.0 is acidic and the lower the figure, the higher the acidity (the greater the hydrogen ion concentration). A solution whose pH is greater than 7.0 is basic or alkaline and the higher the figure, the more basic is the solution.

The body functions within a normal range of 7.35–7.45 pH. This normal range must be maintained by the body systems at all times for the correct internal environment.

## Tissue fluid and the lymphatic system

Each tissue and organ in the body contains a dense network of capillaries (blood vessels that are one cell thick). These are called the *capillary beds*. Tissue fluid is forced under pressure through the capillary walls. This process tends to occur at the artery end of the capillary bed, since blood pressure is greatest at this point.

When tissue fluid is being forced out of the capillaries, the capillary wall acts as a filter holding back red blood cells, most of the white cells and large protein molecules.

Substances which do pass through the capillary wall include:

- Water
- Oxygen
- Glucose
- Fatty acids
- Amino acids
- Vitamins and minerals
- Hormones and enzymes

Tissue fluid flows away from the capillaries and passes among the body cells, which extract oxygen, nutrients and other requirements from it and at the same time release carbon dioxide and other waste materials into it.

### Lymphatic system

This is a system of open-ended tubes within the capillary bed areas, as numerous as the blood capillaries.

*Lymph* is tissue fluid which is not absorbed back into the bloodstream after carrying required substances to the cells. This tissue fluid drains into the open-ended tubes of the lymph system known as *lymph vessels*. The structure of these vessels is similar to that of veins, in that they have a valve system to make sure fluid only flows in one direction . The movement of lymph in these vessels is achieved by the movement of surrounding tissues which squeeze or 'milk' the fluid in the lymph vessels.

At intervals, there are *lymph nodes* (Fig. 2.2), some of which are near the surface (Fig. 2.3). These structures contain a system of narrow channels through

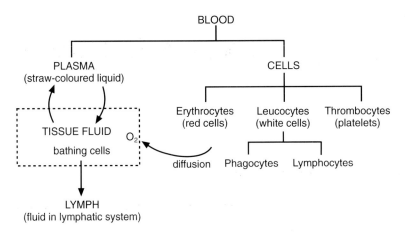

**Fig. 2.5**   Constituents of bood and their functions.

The lymph system is in every sense complementary to the blood and circulation system. Between them, they move fluid and other substances through the tissue spaces and help to keep the internal environment of the body within normal limits for healthy functioning (Figs 2.4 and 2.5).

# Chapter 3
# Body Systems and Functions

## The heart and circulation

This system is part of the transport mechanism of the body. It is made up of:

- A pump – the heart
- A circuit of joined tubes – the arteries, veins and capillaries

Due to the need for a rapid supply of oxygen and nutrients and for the removal of waste substances, the body needs an active supply system. This is provided by the pump, the heart, which is connected to other systems in the body and therefore capable of responding as required to the needs of the tissues.

The circulation connects to all tissues and body cells and will transport:

- *Nutrients* – sugars, fats, amino acids, vitamins, minerals and salts
- *Oxygen*
- *Hormones* – chemical messages controlling the metabolism and development of the body and its operation as a unit
- *White blood cells* – which provide a defence system for the protection of the body

It will also:

- *Provide a clotting mechanism* – to prevent loss of blood from minor damage to the blood vessels
- *Carry heat* – to and from the cells and tissues depending on their requirements
- *Remove waste products* – such as carbon dioxide and other nitrogenous waste like urea and creatinine
- *Carry water* – to replenish the tissues and transport materials in the circulation

### The blood vessels

#### Arteries

- Carry blood away from the heart.
- Carry oxygenated blood (except the pulmonary artery to the lungs).

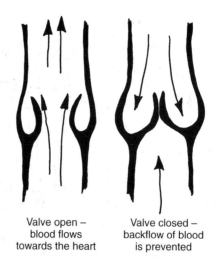

Valve open –
blood flows
towards the heart

Valve closed –
backflow of blood
is prevented

**Fig. 3.1**    Valve system in the veins to prevent backflow of the blood.

- Have thick muscular walls to assist with the movement of blood.
- Under high pressure, from heart muscle contractions.

*Veins*

- Carry blood towards the heart.
- Carry deoxygenated blood (except the pulmonary vein from the lungs to the heart).
- Have thin walls.
- Blood moved under low pressure and by action of surrounding tissues.
- Have a valve system, to prevent backflow of the blood (Fig. 3.1).

*Capillaries*

- Carry blood from artery to vein.
- Blood movement is very slow, to allow maximum diffusion of substances.
- Only one cell thick.
- Connects all cells and tissues, called capillary beds.
- Narrow; may only be wide enough for one blood cell at a time to pass through.

---

**Location names for blood vessels**

The larger blood vessels in the body have a name. For example, the main artery leaving the left side of the heart is called the *aorta*. Whenever the aorta divides to supply an organ, it takes a location name in order to assist anatomists to describe where they are in the body. An example of this would be the aortic division to supply the kidney with blood, called the *renal artery*. When blood leaves the kidney, the vessel is called the *renal vein* and this will rejoin the main vein, the *vena cava*.

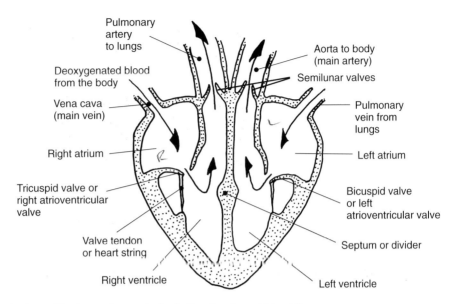

**Fig. 3.2**   The heart. Arrows indicate the direction of blood flow.

## *The heart*

The heart lies between the two sides of the chest (the thorax), surrounded by the lungs, and is held in place by a structure called the *mediastinum* (Fig. 3.2). It is made up of a specialised muscle type which differs from others in three ways:

(1)   Made of branching muscle fibres connected to each other in the form of a network. This enables contractions to begin at one point in the heart and spread outwards in all directions.

(2)   Heart or cardiac muscle contracts and relaxes rhythmically in 'beats'. The rhythm is generated within the muscle itself and not by impulses from the nervous system.

(3)   Heart muscle does not get tired, despite continuous and rapid contractions over many years.

The heart consists of two pumps fused together, each having two chambers:

*   Right atrium and right ventricle
*   Left atrium and left ventricle

The right side of the heart is the less muscular side and pumps deoxygenated blood from the body to the lungs for reoxygenation. The left side of the heart is very muscular and is responsible for pumping oxygenated blood to the body (Fig. 3.3). The blood is under high pressure and this will ensure:

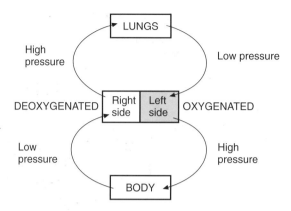

**Fig. 3.3** The heart pump.

- Fast supply of materials to the cells and tissues
- Pushing of fluid from the circulation into the tissues

The heart is surrounded by a thick fibrous bag called the *pericardium*. Blood enters the heart from the body (systemic circulation) via the great veins, the *vena cava*, caudal and cranial vessels. The right atrium contracts to top up the right ventricle. When the right ventricle pumps, it pushes blood out through the pulmonary artery into the lungs (deoxygenated blood). After oxygenation of the blood in the lungs, the blood returns via the pulmonary veins to the left atrium. This contracts to pump the blood through to the left ventricle. The left ventricle is the most muscular chamber of the heart, in order to be able to pump blood around the rest of the body, via the *aorta*.

To stop blood flowing backwards (in the wrong direction), there are valves. On the *right* side of the heart there are the:

- Right atrioventricular valve, also called the tricuspid valve
- Semilunar valve, also called the pulmonary semilunar valve

and on the *left* side of the heart there are the:

- Left atrioventricular valve, also called the bicuspid or mitral valve
- Semilunar valve, also called aortic semilunar valve

At the base of the aorta, just above the semilunar valves, are the entrances to the left and right coronary arteries which supply the *myocardium* (the heart muscles). If these vessels narrow due to fatty deposits or cholesterol, this will reduce the blood flow to the heart muscle, causing lack of oxygen (*ischaemia*) when exercising. This in turn could lead to a heart attack, also called a coronary attack.

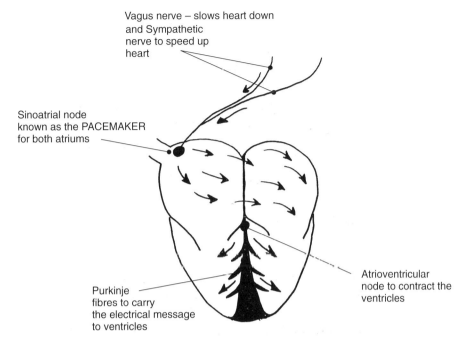

**Fig. 3.4**   Electrical activity during contraction of the heart (pumping). The rhythm for this is provided by the pacemaker.

### Heart beat

Most muscles will contract as a result of impulses reaching them from nerves. The heart is a muscle which beats rhythmically from impulses within its structure. It has special fibres imbedded in the wall of the right atrium called the *sino-atrial node* or, more commonly, the *pacemaker* (Fig. 3.4). This area responds to chemicals like adrenaline or the nervous system command to increase the heart rate in situations of fear, flight or fight.

The electrical message from the pacemaker passes to the right and left atrium, causing them to contract in unison. The impulse then arrives at the atrioventricular node, before passing along special conducting tissue pathways called the *bundles of His*. These fibres lead to the smaller bundles of conducting tissues called *Purkinje fibres*, which cause contraction of the ventricles.

If the pacemaker region of the heart is malfunctioning, the heart rate may fall and not increase with exercise. An animal with this condition will have a slow heart rate with poor exercise tolerance and may faint.

### Heart sounds

There are two sounds:

LUB – DUB

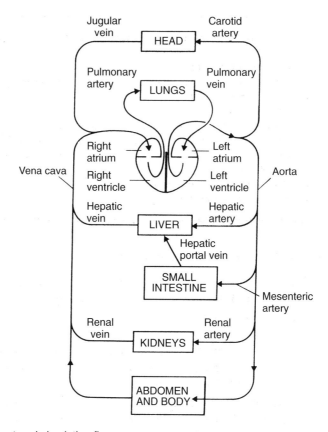

**Fig. 3.5**  Heart and circulation flow.

The first sound, Lub, is produced by the closure of the right and left atrioventricular valves, as the ventricles begin to contract.

When the valves at the base of the aorta and pulmonary artery (semilunar valves) snap shut at the end of the ventricle contraction, then the second sound, Dub, is produced.

If blood within the chest is flowing unevenly or turbulently, a murmur may be detected. This sounds like: Lub – woosh – Dub.

## Respiratory system

Respiration is a term referring to the gaseous exchange between a living structure and its environment.

---

**Structures through which oxygen and carbon dioxide (waste gas) must pass**

*External nares* – nose
*Turbinate bones* – scroll-shaped tubes with epithelial lining in nasal chambers
*Nasopharynx* – back of the throat
*Larynx* – voice box
*Trachea* – open tube for passage of gases only
*Bronchus* – branching of the trachea to the two sides of the chest (thorax)
*Bronchioles* – further branching, getting smaller in diameter
*Alveoli* – air sacs
*Blood capillaries* of the pulmonary system
*Tissue cells* around the body

---

## Characteristics of the respiratory surfaces

Below is a list of features common to all respiratory surfaces. They allow oxygen and carbon dioxide to be exchanged rapidly between an organism and the air which surrounds it.

- Respiratory surfaces have a large surface area to ensure maximum contact with the inhaled air. A mammal's respiratory surface consists of millions of tiny bubble-like air sacs called *alveoli*.
- All respiratory surfaces are moist. This is necessary because oxygen and carbon dioxide can only diffuse in a solution across a respiratory surface (alveoli to blood vessel).
- A respiratory surface is extremely thin, only one cell thick, so that diffusion can take place.
- The inside of a respiratory surface is in contact with a network of capillary blood vessels. This allows gas exchange to take place between the blood and gases.
- There is usually a mechanism which ensures that a respiratory surface is well ventilated, that it receives a steady flow of air. Breathing movements increase the rate of gas exchange by continually removing carbon dioxide and renewing supplies of oxygen to the tissue cells.

## The role of breathing and the circulation

The respiratory and circulatory systems determine how much oxygen and carbon dioxide are present in the body at a given moment. If the amount of oxygen in the blood is low and carbon dioxide high, the body responds by increasing:

- The rate and depth of breathing – ventilation rate.
- The rate at which the heart beats – cardiac frequency.

- The diameter of the arterioles serving those structures that are short of oxygen – vasodilation.

## The respiratory organs of mammals

The thoracic cavity, thorax or chest contains the:

- Heart
- Lungs
- Major blood vessels
- Lymph ducts
- Major nerves

The walls of the thorax are strengthened by the ribs (skeletal system) and caudally (towards the tail) consists of a sheet of muscle called the *diaphragm*. A system of passageways leads from the mouth and nostrils into the lungs and will now be described in more detail (Fig. 3.6).

### The nasal passages

This is where air enters and is warmed to body temperature. The membranes covering the nasal passages also contain the organs responsible for the sense of smell. The walls and base of the nasal passages are lined with a carpet of microscopic hair-like structures called *cilia*. The cilia extend down the trachea to create a surface of moving hairs beating in an upward manner. They help to

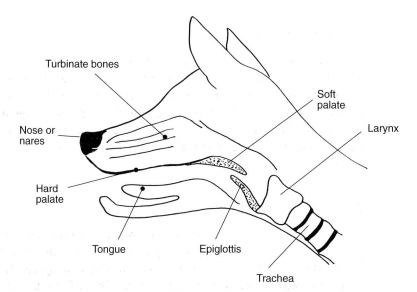

**Fig. 3.6**   Upper respiratory tract.

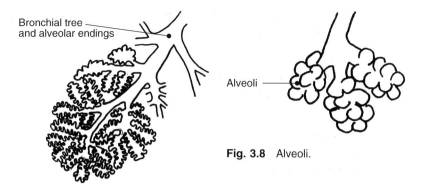

Bronchial tree
and alveolar endings

Alveoli

**Fig. 3.8**   Alveoli.

**Fig. 3.7**   Lung tissue.

expel mucus, which contains dust and micro-organisms which are held in this
thickened liquid.

Air is drawn out of the nasal passages into the pharynx at the back of the
mouth. From here, air is drawn into the trachea via the larynx and past the vocal
cords to activate the voice.

### The bronchial tree

This is the main trunk of the branching trachea, as it supplies lung tissue on both
sides of the thorax. This then becomes the bronchi leading into each lobe of lung
tissue (Fig. 3.7). The bronchi will further divide many times to form a mass of fine
branches called the bronchioles.

### The alveolar ducts

These are the tubes at the end of the bronchioles leading to the air sacs or alveoli
(Fig. 3.8). The alveoli are the respiratory surface of the lungs, giving lung tissue
its spongy appearance. The outer surface of the alveoli is covered by a dense
network of capillary blood vessels. All these capillaries originate from the pulmonary artery (deoxygenated blood) and drain into the pulmonary vein (oxygenated blood) to return to the left side of the heart, for pumping around the
body.

## Gas exchange in the lungs

Blood entering the lungs is deoxygenated because the haemoglobin (red
pigment) in its red cells has given up all its oxygen to the body tissues.

The internal diameter of the lung capillaries is actually smaller than the diameter of the red cells which pass through them. The red cells therefore are squeezed
out of shape as they are forced through the lungs by blood pressure and the speed

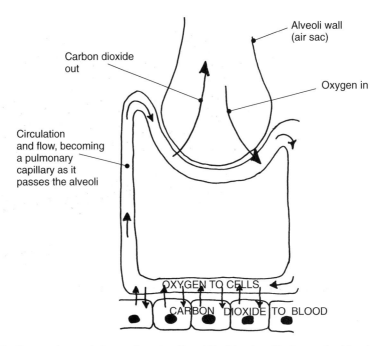

**Fig. 3.9**  Gas exchange between the alveoli and the blood and between the blood and body cells.

at which they move is considerably reduced by the resulting friction. This increases the rate of oxygen absorption in two ways:

(1)   As the red cells squeeze through the narrow capillaries they expose more surface area to the capillary walls, through which oxygen is diffusing and absorbed.
(2)   Their slow rate of progress increases the time available for oxygen to diffuse into the vessels and combine with haemoglobin.

The continuous removal of oxygen as fast as it diffuses into the lung capillaries and the continuous arrival of oxygen in the alveoli owing to breathing movements mean that there is always a higher concentration of oxygen molecules in the alveoli than in the blood. As a result of this, carbon dioxide is exchanged (Fig. 3.9).

### Breathing – ventilation of the lungs

The thorax or pleural cavity is completely airtight and contains a partial vacuum. Its internal pressure is always less than the atmospheric pressure outside the body. The lungs are open to the atmosphere through the trachea and so there is always a higher pressure in the lungs than in the thorax or pleural cavity

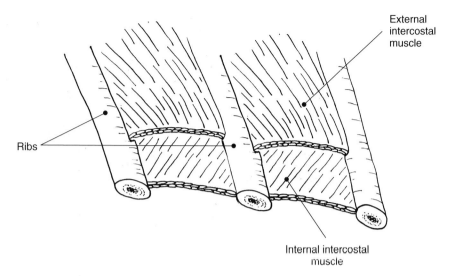

External
intercostal
muscle

Ribs

Internal intercostal
muscle

**Fig. 3.10**   Intercostal muscles and ribs for breathing.

which surrounds them. This pressure difference is extremely important for two reasons:

(1)   The higher pressure in the lungs in relation to the pleural cavity around them stretches the thin elastic alveoli walls so that the lungs as a whole almost fill the thorax on inspiration.
(2)   Since this pressure difference is maintained during breathing movements, when the thoracic cavity increases in size (inspiration), the lungs inflate to fill the extra space available.

At normal atmospheric pressure the above could not happen, hence the need for negative pressure in the thorax.

The muscles which bring about these volume changes are:

•   *The diaphragm* – a dome-shaped sheet of muscle which separates the thorax from the abdomen.
•   *The intercostal muscles* – both internal and external, that cross the gap between each rib and pull the ribs outwards on inspiration (Fig. 3.10).

### Diaphragm

Immediately before inspiration, the diaphragm is dome-shaped and its muscle relaxed. Inspiration takes place when the diaphragm muscle contracts, making the muscle sheet a flatter shape.

*Rib*

At the same time, contraction occurs in the external intercostal muscles between each rib. This increases the size of the rib cage, leading to an increase in lung volume.

- *Inspiration* – the movement of the diaphragm and external intercostal muscles, causing the ribs to move visibly outwards.
- *Expiration* – or breathing out is when the diaphragm and external intercostal muscles relax. This reduces the size of the thorax and the ribs move inwards to the resting position.

Air can be forced out of the lungs by contraction of the internal intercostal muscles but expiration tends to be passive, simply allowing these structures to fall back into the resting position.

## Respiration

The word 'respiration' is derived from the Latin *respirare* which means 'to breathe'. At first, this term referred to the breathing movements which cause air to be drawn into and pushed out of the lungs but now, when defined with strict accuracy, respiration means something entirely different.

---

**The modern definition of respiration**

The processes which lead to, and include, the chemical breakdown of materials to provide energy for life. These processes occur inside the living cells of every type of organism and cause the release of energy from food which is essential for life.

---

Cells cannot use energy as soon as it is released from respiration. This energy is first used to build up a temporary energy store, which takes the form of a chemical called *adenosine triphosphate* or ATP for short. Think of ATP as 'packets' of energy, used to transfer energy from the chemical reactions which release it to the body processes which use it. Respiration fills these ATP packets with energy and they are 'emptied' when energy is needed anywhere in the body.

There are four main advantages to the ATP energy transfer system.

(1)  ATP takes up some energy which would otherwise be lost as heat during the breakdown of glucose by respiratory enzymes.
(2)  Energy is released from ATP the instant it is required without cells having to go through the many different reactions of respiration, allowing for sudden bursts of energy.
(3)  ATP delivers energy in precise amounts.

(4)   Energy can be delivered from ATP to other chemicals without energy loss; for example, from sources of sugars, fats or proteins.

The release of energy at the cellular level is known as the *Krebs cycle*.

## Digestive system

An animal is able to make full use of the food it eats after the following events have taken place, through the digestive tract (Fig. 3.11).

*   Food is first torn up into pieces small enough to swallow (*mastication*).
*   Food enters the alimentary canal mixed with digestive enzymes to further break down the food into simple water-soluble chemicals – the process of *digestion*. It takes place outside the cells of the body.
*   The soluble food then passes through the walls of the gut into the bloodstream. This is called *absorption*.
*   Blood then transports the digested, soluble food to all parts of the body. The food enters cells and is transformed into substances which take part in the body's metabolism. This is called *assimilation*.
*   Any solid substances in food which cannot be digested, like fibres, are expelled from the body as faecal matter or faeces.

### *Foods*

Most foods which animals eat cannot be used by their bodies in the original form for two main reasons:

(1)   Most foods are insoluble and so cannot pass through cell membranes into cells.
(2)   Most foods are chemically different from the substances that make up body tissues. They must therefore be processed before the body can use them by the use of enzymes.

#### Digestive enzymes

All enzymes, whether digestive or belonging to another body system, are *catalysts*. They speed up chemical reactions which would otherwise proceed very slowly. Digestive enzymes are only one example of the many types of enzymes which exist in living animals. The reactions which these enzymes speed up involve splitting complicated molecules into simpler ones.

It is thought that the enzyme combines briefly with molecules of food and while in this state the food undergoes a rapid chemical change in which its molecules are split apart into chemically simpler substances. These substances separate from the enzyme, leaving it immediately available for another identical reaction.

Enzymes are not used up in the reactions which they control but are used countless times in rapid succession.

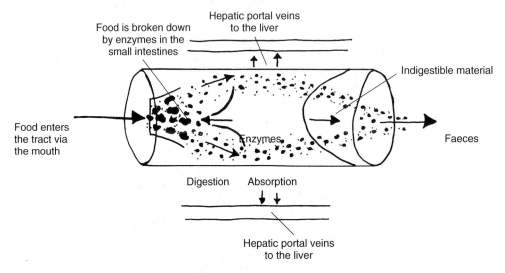

**Fig. 3.11**   Digestive tract – events.

## *Comparative digestive anatomy*

The digestive tract or alimentary canal is simply a continuous tube, with different regions along its length performing different functions.

Anatomically, different species of mammals are grouped according to their digestive anatomy (Figs 3.12 and 3.13).

- Ruminants or polygastric animals (cattle and sheep)
- Simple-stomached animals (e.g. dog, cat and humans)
- Avian (all birds)
- Monogastric herbivores (the horse)

Other definitions may refer to the type of food eaten.

- Carnivores – meat eating
- Omnivores – eat both meat and vegetable matter
- Herbivores – grass eating
- Grainivores – grain eating

The control of digestion of food is both voluntary and involuntary.

- Voluntary
  (a)   Ingestion – placing in mouth
  (b)   Chewing

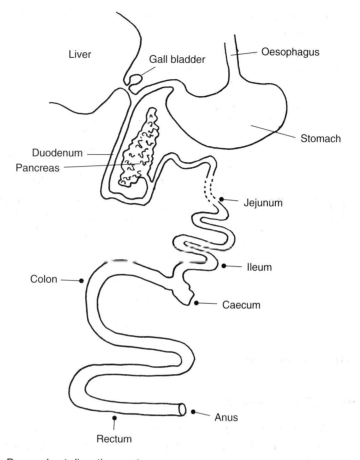

**Fig. 3.12**   Dog and cat digestive anatomy.

    (c)   Swallowing (deglutition)

    (d)   Control of anal sphincter – the muscle controlling the opening and closing of the anus

- Involuntary

    (a)   Opening and closing of sphincters

    (b)   Peristaltic movement (a ripple or wave of muscle) squeezing the food through the gut

    (c)   Release of digestive enzymes

## Digestive tract of dog and cat

- Mouth
- Pharynx
- Oesophagus
- Stomach

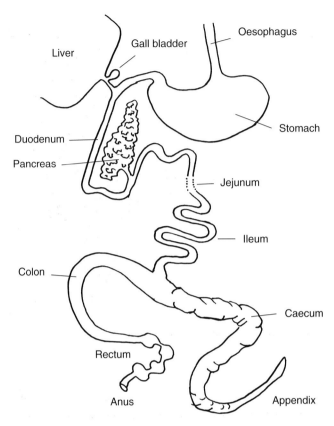

**Fig. 3.13** Rabbit digestive tract showing enlarged caecum and appendix. New food is mixed with caecal (soft) pellets, which are eaten by the rabbit from its own anus (coprophagia).

- Small intestines
    Duodenum
    Jejunum
    Ileum
- Large intestines
    Caecum
    Ascending colon
    Transverse colon
    Descending colon
    Rectum
    Anal canal

*The mouth*

Also called the oral cavity or buccal cavity. The teeth are responsible for grinding, crushing or tearing up the food and with the aid of the tongue and saliva, the food is mixed. The stucture of a basic tooth is shown in Fig. 3.14. Saliva is sup-

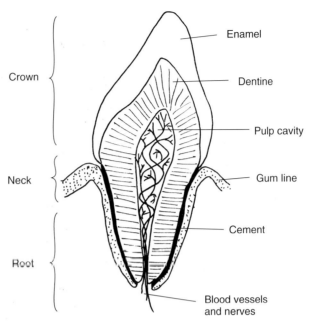

Crown

Neck

Root

Enamel

Dentine

Pulp cavity

Gum line

Cement

Blood vessels
and nerves

**Fig. 3.14**   Structure of the basic tooth.

plied from four glands located around the face. Saliva is usually present in the mouth but its flow is increased by the sight and smell of food. This effect is known as a *gustatory response*. Saliva is made of water with about 1% of it being mucus, electrolytes (salts) and enzymes. The mucus acts as a lubricant and helps in the swallowing of dry food.

The tongue also helps to move the lump of food, known as a *bolus*. The tongue is a mass of striated muscle fibres. It is a sensitive structure with some of the taste buds located on its surface. The tongue has another function, especially in the cat, which is that of grooming.

Fig. 3.15 shows the variation in skulls and dentition in different species.

Common to the digestive and respiratory systems is the *pharynx area*. There are lymphoid areas in the mucous membrane of this area called *tonsils*.

The processes of digestion are shown in Fig. 3.16.

### The oesophagus

Pharyngeal muscles move the food bolus into the oesophagus, which is a simple tube. Swallowing or deglutition is now complete. No digestive enzymes are secreted here but oesophageal cells produce mucus to lubricate the process of peristalsis, the wave-like contraction and relaxation which will propel the food along the tract (Fig. 3.17). These contractions are stimulated by the presence of food.

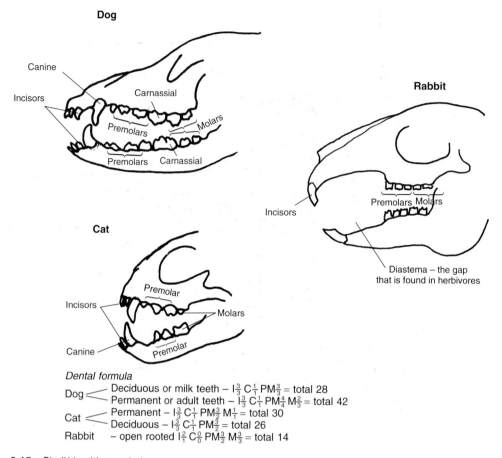

**Dental formula**

Dog $\left\{\begin{array}{l}\text{Deciduous or milk teeth} - I\frac{3}{3}\,C\frac{1}{1}\,PM\frac{3}{3} = \text{total } 28 \\ \text{Permanent or adult teeth} - I\frac{3}{3}\,C\frac{1}{1}\,PM\frac{4}{4}\,M\frac{2}{3} = \text{total } 42\end{array}\right.$

Cat $\left\{\begin{array}{l}\text{Permanent} - I\frac{3}{3}\,C\frac{1}{1}\,PM\frac{3}{2}\,M\frac{1}{1} = \text{total } 30 \\ \text{Deciduous} - I\frac{3}{3}\,C\frac{1}{1}\,PM\frac{2}{2} = \text{total } 26\end{array}\right.$

Rabbit — open rooted $I\frac{2}{1}\,C\frac{0}{0}\,PM\frac{3}{2}\,M\frac{3}{3} = \text{total } 14$

**Fig. 3.15**   Skull/dentition variation.

Enzymes of the digestive tract.

| Secretion | Source | Site of action | Enzyme | Acting on |
|---|---|---|---|---|
| Saliva | Salivary gland | Mouth | Water and mucus | All foods |
| Gastric juice | Stomach | Stomach | Gastrin, pepsin | Protein |
| Bile | Liver | Duodenum | Bile salt | Fats |
| Pancreatic juice | Pancreas | Duodenum | Amylase<br>Trypsin<br>Lipase | Starch<br>Protein<br>Fats |
| Intestinal juice | Intestine wall | Small intestine | Amylase | Starch |

*The cells in the duodenum release the hormone enterokinase, which activates the pancreatic enzymes only when they reach the small intestines. Otherwise they would damage or digest the pancreas.

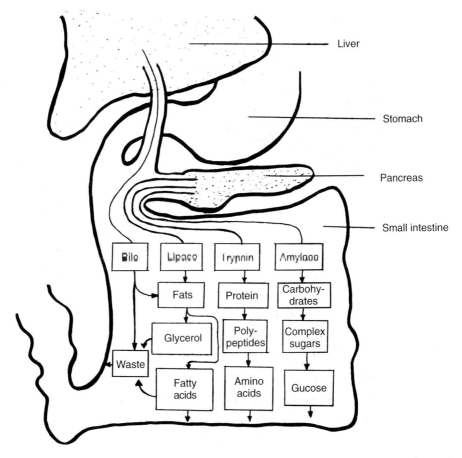

**Fig. 3.16**  The processes of digestion.

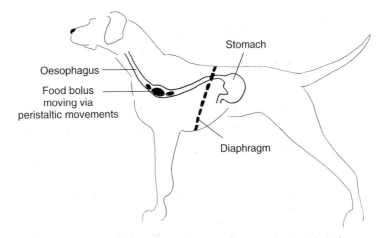

**Fig. 3.17**  Oesophagus and stomach showing food being moved by peristalsis.

### The stomach

The oesophagus enters the stomach via a ring of muscle called the *cardiac sphincter*, a structure which adapts itself to the quantity of food eaten. Some digestion occurs here and the stomach acts as a temporary reservoir. The gastric juices, which contain enzymes and hydrochloric acid, start breaking up the food. The well-mixed and partially digested food, now called *chyme*, is now moved through the sphincter at the stomach exit, called the *pylorus*, and on to the first section of the small intestine.

### The small intestines

So called because of their narrow bore, not their length. Enzyme digestion is completed in the small intestines.

---

- Protein is converted to amino acids
- Fat is converted to fatty acids
- Carbohydrates are converted to simple sugars

---

The chyme is mixed with more enzymes in the first section of the small intestines, the *duodenum*. Some will originate from the duodenum, others from the *pancreas* (its *exocrine* function). The liver also secretes a digestive fluid into the duodenum via the gall bladder; this fluid is ducted into the small intestine to reduce the size of fatty acid molecules and is called *bile*. Bile helps by emulsifying fats and will neutralise the acid fluids from the stomach because it is alkaline.

The second section of the small intestines, called the *jejunum*, continues the mixing and exposing of the chyme to the fluids that reduce it sufficiently for absorption.

The third section of the small intestines is the *ileum*, where the final absorption is completed.

Digestion and absorption are improved by the enormous surface area in the small intestine. Features of this area include:

- The great length of the intestines
- The presence of folds of tissue, increasing the surface area
- The arrangement of finger-like projections called *villi*
- The great number of these villi on the surface of the small intestine, particularly in the final area, the ileum, for maximum absorption

*Absorption.* This takes place via the villi (Fig. 3.18). They contain smooth muscle which allows them to contract and expand. This action brings them into contact with the newly digested food. Simple sugars (mainly glucose) and amino acids

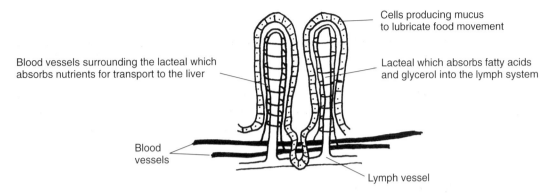

Cells producing mucus
to lubricate food movement

Blood vessels surrounding the lacteal which
absorbs nutrients for transport to the liver

Lacteal which absorbs fatty acids
and glycerol into the lymph system

Blood
vessels

Lymph vessel

**Fig. 3.18**   The villi.

are absorbed, by a combination of diffusion and active transport, across the epithelial lining of the villi into the waiting capillaries beneath. These capillaries drain into the hepatic portal vein which leads to the liver.

Fat is dealt with differently. The fatty acids and glycerol are absorbed into the columnar epithelial cells lining the villi and are pushed into the lymph vessels of the villi as a white emulsion of tiny globules of fat. These globules give the lymph vessels a milky appearance, for which they are known as *lacteals*. The lymph system opens finally into the veins in the thorax and empties via the thoracic duct into the vena cava near the heart.

Salts, vitamins and water are also absorbed in the small intestine.

### The large intestines

This section of intestines is a wider tube and contains no villi. Food materials which are of no value or cannot be broken down to absorbable size are passed from the small to the large intestine through the *ileocaecal valve*. The large intestine in the dog and cat is relatively short in length. Its main purpose is to absorb salt and water. The walls of the colon (large intestine) are much folded for this purpose. By the time materials reach the rectum, indigestible food is in a semi-solid condition ready to be voided through the anus as faeces.

The first part of the large intestines is called the *caecum*. It is a blind-ended sac which has no function in carnivores but is enlarged in herbivores as a site of bacterial breakdown of vegetable food matter.

The colon is divided into three sections:

- Ascending
- Transverse
- Descending

The colon terminates in the rectum area, where waste products are held before excretion as faecal material.

The last part of the tract is closed by sphincter muscles and is known as the anal canal, over which the animal has control via skeletal muscle (voluntary muscle). Defecation involves relaxation of the anal sphincter but diarrhoea or illness may override this control. Diarrhoea is defined as the frequent evacuation of watery faeces. If defecation is delayed too long, constipation may result.

Consistent with its functions of water absorption and faecal movement, the large intestine is lined with a mucus-secreting surface. This assists in the movement of materials by a lubricating action. The mucus prevents the total drying out of the faeces, which might then damage the lining.

---

**Brief summary of digestion and absorption of the main food constituents**

- *Proteins* – come from muscle meat, egg or vegetable proteins like soya bean. These are broken down in the stomach and small intestines to become amino acids and absorbed into the bloodstream for transport to the liver, where they are processed.
- *Carbohydrates* – are found as cereals like biscuit potatoes or pasta. They are broken down into simple sugars (*glucose*) and absorbed into the bloodstream for transport to the liver where they may be stored as *glycogen*. When required by the body for energy, glycogen can be turned back into glucose.
- *Fats* – are found as animal fat or vegetable oils and are broken down into fatty acids and glycerols by bile and enzymes in the small intestines. Most will enter the lacteals in the villi to travel via the lymph system, finally reaching the bloodstream for use or storage.

---

# Liver and pancreas

The liver is the largest organ of the body, situated immediately caudal to the diaphragm in the abdomen. About 75% of the liver's blood supply comes from the hepatic portal system of vessels (Fig. 3.19). This ensures that the products of digestion are absorbed into the bloodstream and travel to the liver for processing, before moving on either to storage or to be used in another way. The remaining 25% of blood to the liver arrives via the hepatic artery.

The special cells that make up the liver are called *hepatocytes*. The liver is a very complex chemical factory which produces materials for use within the body from the products of digestion which come directly to it from the gut.

## Functions of the liver

It is thought that the liver performs over 500 functions. The main functions are as follows:

- Regulation of sugar which has four possible fates:
  (1)   used as energy source (Krebs cycle)

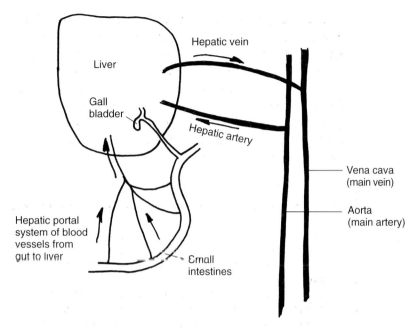

**Fig. 3.19**   Blood supply to the liver.

(2)   stored as glycogen in the liver
(3)   converted to fat and stored around the body
(4)   passed directly into the circulation
- Regulation of lipids (fats)
- Regulation of amino acids and proteins
- Heat production
- Bile production
- Formation of cholesterol
- Elimination of sex hormones
- Storage and filtration of blood
- Elimination of haemoglobin from exhausted red blood cells
- Formation of urea to be passed on to the kidneys for removal from the body
- Creation of plasma proteins (synthesis)
- Storage of vitamins A, D and $B_{12}$ and minerals like iron and copper

### The pancreas

The pancreas is a large grey-pink gland, which lies in the abdomen close to the stomach and the duodenum section of the small intestine. It is made up of two parts which are joined together, giving the pancreas its boomerang shape.

There are two types of tissue present within the gland and these have very different functions.

- *Exocrine tissue* – which produces digestive enzymes
- *Endocrine tissue* – which produces hormones like insulin to help in controlling sugar in the body.

# Urinary system

This system has several functions but its main one is that of excretion and removal of waste products from the body. Wastes are toxic if allowed to accumulate so this removal of harmful materials, which are the end products of metabolism, is essential and continuous.

**Functions include:**

- loss or conservation of body water
- excretion of unwanted substances or those in excess to requirements
- storage of products before their removal from the body
- endocrine organ producing hormones.

The mammalian urinary tract consists of:

- Two kidneys
- Two ureters
- One bladder
- One urethra

## The kidneys

These are bean shaped and situated one on each side of the abdomen (Fig. 3.20). Each contains specialised cells which filter out materials which must be removed from the body and conserve those which the body needs. These cells are called the *nephrons*, from which we get the term *nephritis*, meaning inflammation of the kidney nephron cells.

The blood supply to the kidneys is via the renal artery directly from the aorta and drains away from the kidney via the renal vein directly into the vena cava.

## The nephron

This is the special cell of the urinary system. The structure is as follows (Fig. 3.21):

- *Glomerulus* – a network or knot of artery from branches of the renal artery in the cortex section of the kidney.

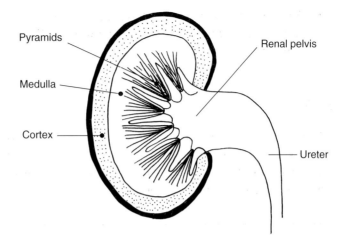

**Fig. 3.20**  The kidney.

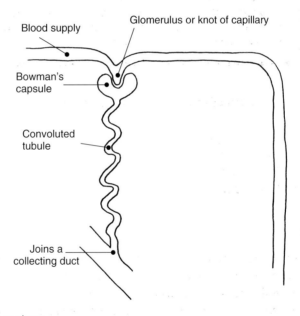

**Fig. 3.21**  The nephron.

- *Bowman's capsule* – the cup-shaped part of the nephron, at the start of the tubule. It is into this that the glomerulus fits and contacts, resulting in the start of blood filtration and the removal of urea and other nitrogenous wastes.
- *Proximal tubule* – the start of the long tube through which the filtered substances will pass.
- *Loop of Henle and distal tubule* – this is where, on instruction from hormones, the nephron conserves water, salts and sugars or, if the body has an excess, it is instructed to add the excess to the forming urine for removal from the body.

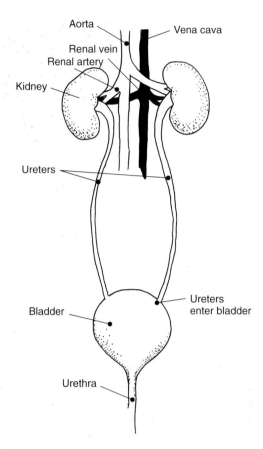

Aorta
Vena cava
Renal vein
Renal artery
Kidney
Ureters
Ureters
enter bladder
Bladder
Urethra

**Fig. 3.22** The urinary system.

The distal tubule joins a collecting duct which directs the urine to the pelvis region of the kidney, where all nephrons drain, then along the ureter to the bladder for temporary storage. When the bladder is full, the animal receives this information from the brain and relaxes the sphincter muscle from the bladder to the urethra and the outside (Fig. 3.22). The act of passing urine is called *micturition*.

## Nervous system

The nervous system provides the quickest means of communication within the body. Information is received both from outside the animal (the environment) and from inside the animal's body. The response to information received has to be co-ordinated in order for the body systems to unite in their response, to produce the desired effect.

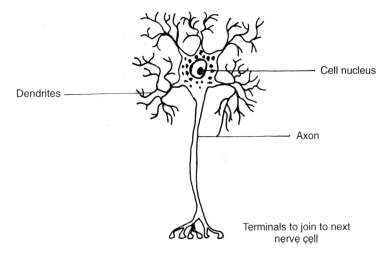

Cell nucleus

Dendrites

Axon

Terminals to join to next
nerve cell

**Fig. 3.23**  Nerve cell – the neurone.

Messages to the body are carried in two ways:

(1)  *Electrical* – these are impulses which travel along the nerves and give fast
     response to a situation or stimulus (nervous system). The electrical messages
     stimulate movement of muscles:
     (a)  cardiac – the heart
     (b)  skeletal – bones and joints
     (c)  involuntary – organs and tissues.
(2)  *Chemical* – these are hormones which, once released into the bloodstream,
     will travel more slowly to their target organ. The body response is seen after
     a period of time (endocrine system).

Body co-ordination by nervous system tissue is conducted by the nerve cells,
the *neurones* (Fig. 3.23), together with various forms of supporting tissue in which
they are embedded. These cells are the basic functional unit of the nervous system
and are found in bundles, called *nerves*.

There are four types of neurone.

(1)  *Sensory* – those attached to the senses, like sight, hearing, taste, smell and
     touch. These carry messages about information outside the body to the
     brain.
(2)  *Relay* – information or messages between neurones.
(3)  *Motor* – these link up to relay neurones and with muscle or gland cells in
     order to deliver messages from the central nervous system (brain and spinal
     cord) to initiate an action. This may be the release of more hormone or the
     movement of a muscle.

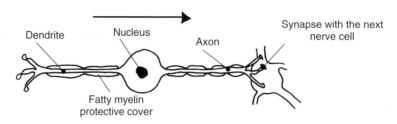

**Fig. 3.24**   Nerve cell and direction of electrical impulse.

(4)   *Network* – these link the cell branches in order to keep the information and action by the brain and spinal cord networked like a computer.

The shape of the nerve cell will vary to suit the tissue into which it links but the basic components remain the same.

- A cell body containing the nucleus.
- Cell processes which lead to and from the cell body (Fig. 3.24):
    (a)   the *axon* – which carries the impulses away from the cell body
    (b)   the *dendrite* – which carries impulses towards the cell body.

The property of a nerve cell is that its cell membrane is electrically charged by the action of *ions* (salts or electrolytes) such as potassium or sodium. Although the voltage carried is small, when discharged along the length of nerves, it allows the system to act as a high-speed electrical signalling system. After the signal, the membrane is recharged and returns to a resting position, awaiting the next signal.

The junction between two or more neurones is called a *synapse* (Fig. 3.25). Electrical impulses cannot pass across this gap, so communication is dependent upon a chemical transmitter substance – a *neurotransmitter*. This substance will connect two neurones for less than one millisecond, allowing the impulse to pass on. The chemical is then destroyed by another substance and recreated again before each future impulse.

### Reflex action or arc (Fig. 3.26)

This refers to an automatic and very rapid response to a potentially harmful stimulus which is usually external to the body. It is a survival response.

The structural basis of reflex action is the *reflex arc*, which represents the series of units of nerve tissue through which impulses have to pass in order to bring about a reflex response. The sensory tissues receiving the information are called *receptors* and may be scattered sensory cells in the skin or special sense receptors like the eye or ear. Their stimulation results in impulses being generated in

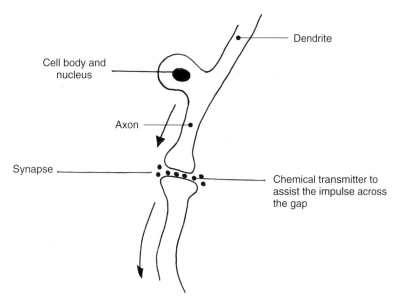

**Fig. 3.25** A synapse – the junction between two or more neurones.

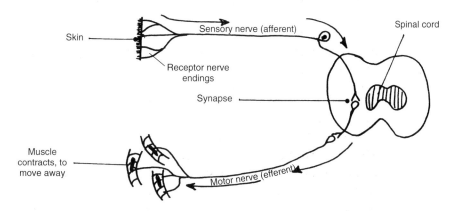

**Fig. 3.26** Reflex arc.

sensory (*afferent*) neurones located in the peripheral nerves (on or near the body surface). These afferent neurones take the impulse to the central nervous system (only to the spinal cord) where a connection nerve in the cord connects to a motor (*efferent*) neurone. This will take the impulse or message to an effector tissue like a gland or to a muscle for the desired effect – survival.

The common example used is touching a hot surface, when the reflex arc ensures that the animal suffers minimal harm as the foot is speedily withdrawn from the danger.

### *Central nervous system*

Made up of the brain and spinal cord.

#### The brain

The general function of the brain is to co-ordinate the body's activities. It receives all sensory information and processes it for:

- Immediate use – reflex arc.
- Later use – storing it in memory, passing orders via neurones and hormones, constantly monitoring the internal body systems for any change.

The brain is divided into three parts (Fig. 3.27).

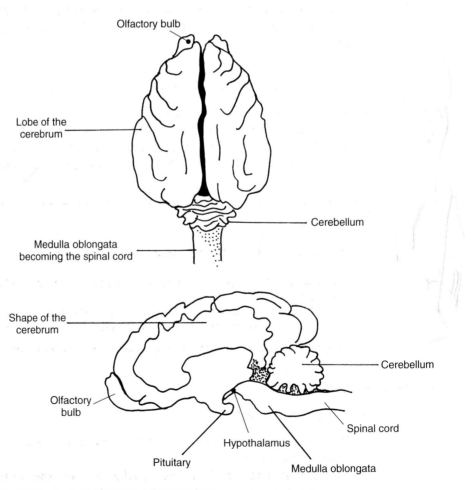

**Fig. 3.27**  Parts of the brain, from two views.

(1) *Forebrain* – cerebrum, divided into two areas called the cerebral hemispheres (including the hypothalamus), involved with voluntary movement and the senses.
(2) *Midbrain* – involved with sight, hearing, muscle control and body position.
(3) *Hindbrain* – the cerebellum, the pons and the medulla oblongata. Involved with complicated movements of the body, control of the circulation and respiration and awareness of surroundings.

### The spinal cord

The cord extends from the base of the skull to the lumbar/sacral region of the spine, over the pelvis. It is a continuation of the hindbrain and medulla oblongata. The cord is protected by the *vertebrae* and the *meninges*. The canal, which runs through each vertebra, houses the spinal cord

The cord divides into many branching spinal nerves. This continues first inside the vertebrae, then on the outside of the coccygeal vertebrae as the *cauda equina* (resembling a horse's tail), to supply motor and sensory nerves to the tip of the animal's tail.

### Protection of the brain and spinal cord

- *Bones* – skull and bones of the spine.
- *Meninges* – the three membranes, in turn separated by the cerebrospinal fluid.
- *Blood–brain barrier* – a mechanism located in a continuous layer of endothelial cells which allows only useful substances to enter the brain.

---

**Meninges**

The three protective membranes covering the brain and spinal cord

- *Dura mater* – the tough outer membrane, in contact with the bone of the skull and the vertebrae.
- *Arachnoid* – a fine network of collagen and elastic fibres, next to the dura mater.
- *Pia mater* – the membrane in contact with the brain and spinal cord tissue surface.

---

## Peripheral nervous system

### Voluntary nervous system

- Paired spinal nerves containing both sensory and motor fibres, forming a mixed spinal nerve.
- Twelve cranial nerves. These are mixed nerves and can contain motor and sensory, voluntary and autonomic fibres (Table 3.2).

**Table 3.2** The 12 cranial nerves.

| Number | Name | Type | Function |
|---|---|---|---|
| I | Olfactory | Sensory | Smell |
| II | Optic | Sensory | Vision, pupil light response |
| III | Oculomotor | Motor | Eye movement, pupil constriction |
| IV | Trochlear | Motor | Eye movement |
| V | Trigeminal | Mixed | Mastication, touch and pain receptors |
| VI | Abducens | Motor | Eye movement |
| VII | Facial | Mixed | Salivation, facial expression, taste |
| VIII | Auditory/ vestibulocochlear | Sensory | Hearing, balance |
| IX | Glossopharyngeal | Mixed | Taste, laryngeal muscles |
| X | Vagus | Mixed | Vocalisation, swallowing Decrease in heart rate Abdominal organs |
| XI | Accessory | Motor | Head movement |
| XII | Hypoglossal | Motor | Tongue movement |

*Involuntary or autonomic nervous system*

- Sympathetic nervous system
- Parasympathetic nervous system

The involuntary or autonomic nervous system is not under conscious control and is involved with the regulation of body functions. It is divided into two parts, distinguished by their function and by the chemical transmitters (neurotransmitters) used at the synapse between nerve cells.

**Sympathetic system**

Chemical – adrenaline
Prepares body for fight, fright and flight
Inhibits salivation
Increases heart rate
Increases respiratory rate

**Parasympathetic system**

Chemical – cholinesterase
Assists in day-to-day function of the body
Stimulates salivation
Decreases heart rate back to normal
Decreases respiratory rate

# Endocrine system

This is made up of a system of ductless glands which are sites for the production of hormones (Fig. 3.28). The hormones are discharged directly into the blood for circulation to the target organ or tissue. Hormones are sometimes referred to as chemical messengers.

The word 'endocrine' means 'internal secretion' and the organs of this system are therefore glands of internal secretion. Although the glands are sited all over the body, they influence one another and, through their interactions, are integrated into a highly co-ordinated system.

The messages from the hormones:

- Have long-lasting effects on their targets (hours to days)
- Assist in the constant adjustment of the internal body
- Arrive at their target at the speed of the circulating blood

The nervous and endocrine systems are linked. The endocrine gland that controls the functions of all the other glands in this system, the pituitary or master gland, is in the brain close to the hypothalamus.

## The glands

### Pituitary

Controlling the other glands, body growth and the internal body, the pituitary is situated at the base of the brain. It is divided into two parts.

The *anterior* pituitary produces:

- Thyrotropic or thyroid-stimulating hormone (TSH) for production of thyroid hormone.
- Adrenocorticotropic hormone (ACTH) for control of adrenal glands and release of corticosteroids.
- Growth hormone or somatotropin (GH) which promotes the body's growth.
- Gonadotropins which influence the ovaries and testes:
  - (a) follicle-stimulating hormone (FSH) promotes the ripening of the eggs in the ovaries and the secretion of oestrogen in the female. In the male, FSH assists the development of the sperm cells
  - (b) luteinizing hormone (LH) stimulates ovulation and the secretion of oestrogen and progesterone in the female. In the male, it stimulates the development and release of testosterone
  - (c) prolactin or lactogenic hormone develops mammary tissues during pregnancy for milk production.

The *posterior pituitary* produces:

- Antidiuretic hormone (ADH) or vasopressin, which prevents excessive loss of water from the body via the kidneys.
- Oxytocin which stimulates the release of milk and uterine contractions during parturition.

### Thyroid

This gland regulates growth, body development and metabolism. It is located below the larynx near the trachea. It produces and secretes the thyroid hormone which regulates metabolism, growth and development.

### Parathyroid

The parathyroid gland is situated near the thyroid gland. It produces parathyroid hormone which regulates the calcium and phosphorus levels in the blood and bones.

### Adrenals

The adrenals regulate growth of bones, muscle development and secondary sex characteristics. These two small glands are located near the kidneys. The glands are divided into:

- *Cortex* – producing steroids, which are concerned with the regulation of sodium and potassium and the body water (fluids) balance. An example of a hormone produced here is aldosterone. Corticosteroids produced assist in the metabolism of nutrients, antibody formation and dealing with stress. Also produced here are the hormones responsible for the male and female sex characteristics.
- *Medulla* – secretes adrenaline and noradrenaline, which prepare the body for flight or fight in stressful situations.

### Pancreas

The pancreas regulates the use and storage of glucose in the body and is considered a part of the digestive system. It lies close to the stomach in a loop of the small intestine (duodenum). It produces insulin for the use and storage of simple sugars from the breakdown of carbohydrates in the diet.

### Pineal gland

This is a small oval gland situated near the base of the brain. It secretes melatonin, which inhibits gonad activity. The secretions may be linked to seasonal light levels, which control timing of an animal's oestrus cycle.

### Gonads

Female (ovaries) and male (testes) gonads produce hormones for the functioning of the reproductive systems of each sex.

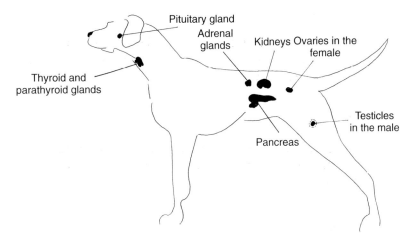

**Fig. 3.28**   Endocrine glands in the dog.

- *Ovaries* – produce some of the oestrogen hormone responsible for the secondary sex characteristics and oestrus cycles. They also produce progesterone for the preparation of the uterus in pregnancy.
- *Testes* – produce testosterone, responsible for male secondary sex characteristics.

The following organs are not endocrine glands but do produce hormones.

- *Kidney* – produces the hormone erythropoietin, which stimulates the production of red cells in active bone marrow sites.
- *Intestines* – produce hormones to promote the production of digestive enzyme compounds from organs such as the pancreas.

## Sense organs

Sense organs collect stimuli. However, sensations are interpreted by the brain once it is fed the information via nerves. Sense organs collect information from inside and outside the body.

### Inside the body

- Temperature monitored by the hypothalamus of the brain.
- Regulation of breathing by measuring the carbon dioxide levels.
- Tension of muscles or tendons which prevents overexercise and damage.

### Outside the body

- Light, dark, shape or colour becomes sight.
- Sound and changes of body position become hearing and balance.

- Airborne chemicals become smells.
- Ingested chemicals become tastes.
- Touch, heat and cold pass survival information to the brain.

### The eye

This is the organ of vision (Fig. 3.29). The eye resembles a camera in at least three ways:

(1)  Both focus light. In the eye the apparatus for this consists of the transparent cornea and lens. These act like the glass lens of the camera in forming the image.
(2)  This image falls on a layer of receptors called the *retina* which, like the film in a camera, is sensitive to light.
(3)  Eyes and cameras have a mechanism called an *iris diaphragm*, which is an opaque disc with a hole at the centre. This increases or decreases in size to control light entering the eye.

The retina transforms light into a stream of nerve impulses which pass down the optic nerve to the brain, to form a picture. The frequency and pattern of these impulses vary according to patches of colour, light and shade which make up the retinal image. The visual area of the brain interprets these impulses to form moving impressions.

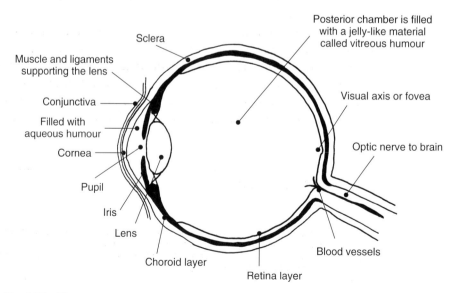

**Fig. 3.29**  The eye.

*Protection of the eyes*

- Cavities in the skull called the *orbits* protect the eye ball with a bone and cartilage ring.
- The transparent, self-repairing skin on the eye called the conjunctiva.
- Tears keep the eyes moist; a stream of liquid from the tear glands is wiped across the eye by blinking and prevents the tissues from becoming too dry.
- The blink reflex to guard against dust and other objects which might enter the eye socket.

*Nourishment and support tissues of the eye*

The eye receives oxygen via blood vessels which enter with the optic nerve, at the back of the eye. These vessels spread out through the *choroid layer* and over the surface of the *retina*.

The *cornea* and *lens* obtain oxygen and food by diffusion from vessels in the liquid in the front chamber of the eye – the *aqueous humour*.

*Vitreous humour* is a jelly in the back cavity of the eye which helps to maintain the shape of the eye.

The *iris* is the coloured part of the eye and has a round hole in its centre called the *pupil*. The iris consists of muscles which radiate out and contract to enlarge the size of the pupil and circular muscles, which make it smaller in size. The iris regulates the amount of light reaching the retina.

The lens consists of layers of transparent material arranged like the skins of an onion, which are enclosed in an elastic outer membrane. These are held in place by *suspensory ligaments*, which in turn are attached to a ring of muscle called the *ciliary muscle*.

The retina is covered with light-sensitive receptors called *rods and cones* (due to their shape). These are buried under nerve fibres and a layer of blood capillaries which conduct the impulses to the brain. These layers are absent from the area where the clearest image is formed, the *fovea*. This area is directly opposite the lens and is the most sensitive part of the eye for colour vision.

The retina contains an area called the *blind spot* (Fig. 3.30). It consists of blood

---

**Detecting the blind spot**

+                                                    ●

Hold this page with the cross and spot at arm's length. Close the left eye and stare at the cross with the right eye. Note that the black circle is still visible.
Bring the page slowly towards the face. At a certain point the circle will disappear. This happens when its image falls on the blind spot.

---

**Fig. 3.30**  Detecting the eye's blind spot.

vessels and nerve fibres leading to the optic nerve. Due to these tissues this area is completely insensitive to light.

## The ear

The anatomy of the ear is shown in Fig. 3.31. Functions are:

- Hearing
- Detecting change in body position
- Balance

The ear is divided into three sections:

(1)  *Outer* – for sound gathering.
(2)  *Middle* – transmits vibrations to the oval window of the inner ear.
(3)  *Inner* – receives the sound waves, passes them to the nerve that connects to the brain for conversion into hearing.

### Outer ear

This is made up of the earflap or *pinna* and the canal. The shape of the canal will vary between species and breeds. This part of the ear collects sound waves and

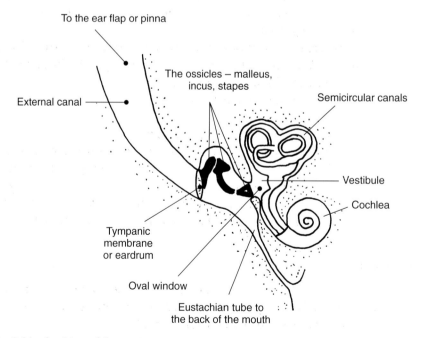

**Fig. 3.31**  Anatomy of the ear.

directs them into the canal, which is lined with modified sebaceous glands. These glands produce wax, as a protective layer. The canal leads to the eardrum or *tympanic membrane*.

### Middle ear

This lies beyond the eardrum in the tympanic cavity, which is made of bone, on the ventral surface of the skull. The cavity contains three small bones called *ossicles*.

* *Malleus* – known as the hammer (contacts the eardrum)
* *Incus* – known as the anvil
* *Stapes* – known as the stirrup (contacts the oval window)

Vibrations of the eardrum (tympanic membrane) are transmitted by these bones to the *oval window*, which is the junction between the middle and inner ear.

The link between the middle ear and the throat/pharynx is the *auditory tube* (*Eustachian tube*). This tube allows air pressure to be equalised on either side of the eardrum.

### Inner ear

This is situated in the temporal bone of the skull. It is here that sound vibrations are converted into nervous impulses and the inner ear is also involved in maintaining balance.

This area consists of a closed system of delicate tubes, called the *membranous labyrinth*, which contains a fluid caued *endolymph*. The labyrinth is itself bathed in a separate fluid, the *perilymph*.

The labyrinth is made up of:

* The *vestibule* – a sac-like structure.
* The *semicircular canals* – these are three loops at right angles to each other. They respond to movement of the endolymph, the angle of the head and changes in body position.
* The *cochlea* – a snail-shaped structure responsible for converting sound waves into nerve impulses which are converted in the brain to hearing.

## Other senses

*Smell* or olfaction is important for the selection of food and scenting other animals. Olfactory membranes can also receive stimuli from the mouth so as a result, taste is sometimes actually smell.

*Taste* or gustation arises from taste cells contained in the mucous membranes of the mouth and on the base of the tongue. Taste and smell will stimulate salivation and the digestive tract in readiness for food to be swallowed.

*Jacobson's organ*, or the vomeronasal organ, supplements the sense of smell in receiving pheromone information about other animals. It is involved in the location of an animal on heat for reproductive purposes.

## Skin or integument

The anatomy of the skin is shown in Fig. 3.32.

### *Function*

- *Protection* – from the external environment and the controlled internal environment of the body, actively preventing:
  (a)  water loss
  (b)  absorption of toxic or harmful substances
  (c)  entry of disease-producing micro-organisms (*pathogens*).
- *Production* – of vitamin D which is required for the absorption of calcium from the intestines.
- *Sense organ* – receptor nerves throughout the skin's surface respond to:
  (a)  touch
  (b)  temperature
  (c)  pressure
  (d)  pain.

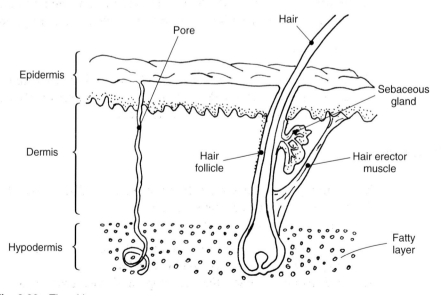

**Fig. 3.32**  The skin.

- *Storage* – of fat as adipose tissue. This is a body energy store and acts as an insulation layer to help maintain body temperature in cold weather.
- *Temperature control*
  (a) For heat loss:
    - vasodilation of surface blood vessels (widening of the vessel wall)
    - sweating.
  (b) For heat gain:
    - vasoconstriction of blood vessels (narrowing of the vessel wall)
    - erection of surface hair/coat/feathers to trap a layer of air for insulation
    - a fat layer under the skin (*subcutaneous layer*).
- *Scent gland* – for communication with other animals for reproductive purposes (production of pheromones) or territorial purposes (use of the anal glands on either side of the anus).

### Structure

- *Epidermis* – is the outer layer, which is hard and dry and contains no blood vessels. This layer continually looses dead cells.
- *Dermis* – is the layer below the epidermis and is a type of connective tissue containing nerves, blood vessels, glands and hair roots.
- *Hypodermis* – is the innermost layer of the skin.

#### Hair

This covers most of an animal's surface area. It is made of *keratin* (a protein made by the body) and pigments for colour. It grows from the hair *follicle* and attached to the deepest section of the hair is the smooth (involuntary) muscle called the *erector pili* muscle which is responsible for moving the hair upright.

#### Sweat glands

Sweat or sebaceous glands produce *sebum* which will include a pheromone. Other very specialised glands in the skin include mammary glands for milk production and anal glands for scenting territory.

## Skeleton

The anatomy of the skeleton is shown in Fig. 3.33a. Figs 3.33b and c show the differences between dog and cat skeletons.

The skeleton is divided into three parts:

(1) *Axial* – skull, vertebral column (spine), ribs and sternum.
(2) *Appendicular* – the fore and hind limbs.
(3) *Splanchnic* – bones that develop in tissues, such as the os penis and fabellae.

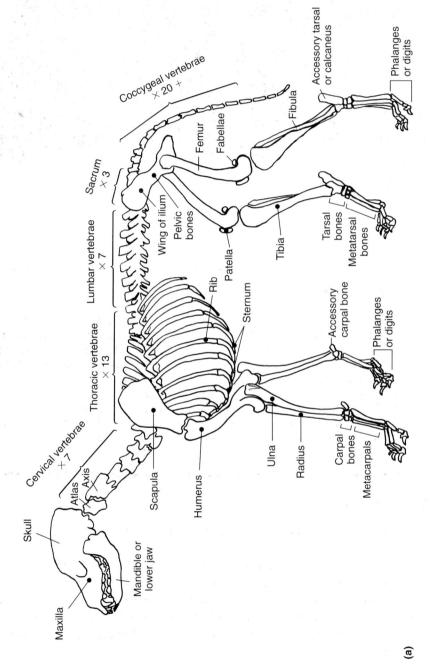

(a)

**Fig. 3.33** (a) Anatomy of the skeleton.

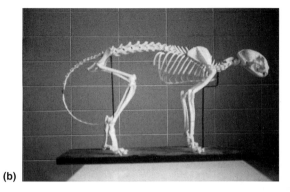

(b)

**Fig. 3.33**  Skeleton of cat.

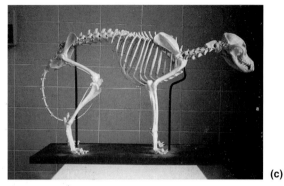

(c)

**Fig. 3.33**  Skeleton of dog.

**Position terms**

- *Proximal* – meaning 'nearer to the centre of the body' (for example, the part of the femur bone closest to the hip joint would be called the proximal end of femur).
- *Distal* – meaning 'further from the centre of the body' (for example, the part of the femur bone nearest to the knee or stifle would be called the distal end of femur).
- *Cranial* – descriptive term meaning 'towards or within the head'.
- *Dorsal* – the surface of the body which is on top.
- *Caudal* – a descriptive term meaning 'towards or within the tail'.
- *Medial* – a term describing something that lies nearest to the midline of the body.
- *Ventral* – any surface of the body that is facing the ground.
- *Lateral* – the sides of the body, both left and right.

## *Movements of the body*

These are movements of a whole limb relative to the body.

- *Protraction* – movement of a limb towards the head (cranially).
- *Retraction* – movement of a limb towards the tail (caudally).
- *Elevation* – movement of a limb up and nearer the body (proximal to body).
- *Adduction* – movement of a limb towards the middle of the body (midline).
- *Abduction* – movement of a limb away from the middle of the body (away from the midline).

## *Bone structure*

Bone is hard and to some extent also flexible (Fig. 3.34). The cells in bone are arranged as cylinders and in layers in order to give bone its strength. They also

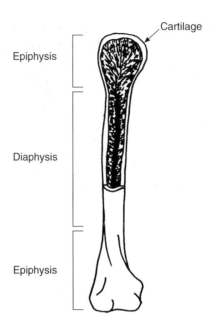

**Fig. 3.34**  Bone structure.

secrete minerals like calcium and phosphorus, which provide its rigid nature. The structure of bones provides for the maximum resistance to mechanical stresses, while maintaining the least bony mass.

Bone is made of two types of cells.

- *Osteoblasts* are responsible for the secretion of material which, when mineralised, will become bone. Osteoblasts become trapped in the forming bone and are then called *osteocytes*.
- *Osteoclasts* are responsible for reabsorbing materials and therefore for the remodelling of bone.

In the general structure of long bones, there are two types of bone materials.

- *Compact* bone which will form the dense walls of the bone shaft.
- *Cancellous* or *spongy* bone which is found in the central medullary cavity. As the name suggests, this bone consists of a network and spaces all linked to each other.

The *medullary cavity* of most bones contains active or red marrow which is responsible for the production of platelets, red and white blood cells. The yellow, rather fatty-looking material sometimes is found in the medullary cavities is inactive bone marrow.

The outer surface of bone is covered with a layer of dense fibrous connective tissue called the *periosteum* into which are inserted muscles, tendons and ligaments for attachment. The inner surface of bone is covered by a delicate connective tissue layer, called the *endosteum*. Both these layers contain cells, which assist in the remodelling and repair of bone if it becomes damaged.

The function of bone and the skeletal system is to:

- Support the body
- Provide levers for movement
- Protect organs
- Maintain mineral levels in the body
- Produce blood cells (both red and white)

### Joints

These are the articular surfaces of the ends of bones, always protected by a layer of cartilage (hyaline). The study of joints is termed *arthrology*. When joints become inflamed, this is termed *arthritis*.

Joints are places where different bones come into anatomical contact with each other.

- *Synarthroses* – are joints which are immovable, e.g. joints of the skull.
- *Diarthroses* – are joints where movement of adjacent bones can occur and these are usually related to the limbs, e.g. synovial joints.
- *Amphiarthroses* – are joints which share some of the characteristics of the synarthroses and diarthroses but have limited movement, e.g. between the vertebrae of the spine.

Joints are further commonly classified as:

- *Fibrous* – no movement at all. Also called suture joints, such as the bones of the skull.
- *Cartilaginous* – some movement to these. Examples are found where there are right and left sides, e.g. the lower jaw (mandibles) and in the pelvis.
- *Synovial* (Fig. 3.35) – plenty of movement to these joints. They also have other features:
  (a)  cartilage surfaces at bone ends
  (b)  joint membrane or capsule
  (c)  joint fluid for lubricatation (synovial fluid).

Synovial joints may be called *simple* joints if they contain two articular surfaces, an example being the two bones which make up the shoulder joint. *Compound* joints have more than two articular surfaces, as in the elbow where three bones come together to form the joint.

The following simple and compound joints are generally recognised.

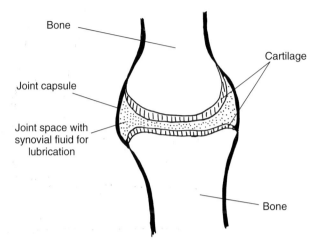

**Fig. 3.35**   Simple synovial joint.

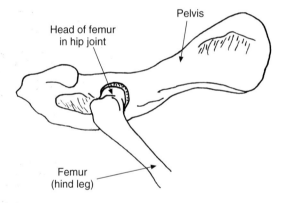

**Fig. 3.36**   Ball and socket joint.

- Ball and socket (femur/acetabulum) (Fig. 3.36)
- Hinge (humerus/radius and ulna) (Fig. 3.37)
- Pivot (radius/ulna or atlas/axis) (Fig. 3.38)
- Saddle (between phalanges or toes) (Fig. 3.39)
- Plane or gliding (between carpals/tarsals) (Fig. 3.39)
- Condylar (stifle or knee)

The stability of all synovial joints is improved by:

- Ligaments
- Surrounding muscles and tendons
- Well-shaped/fitting articular bone surfaces

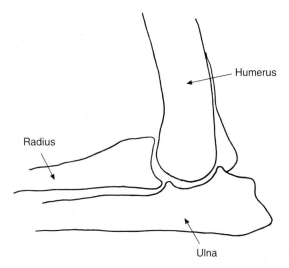

**Fig. 3.37** Hinge joint.

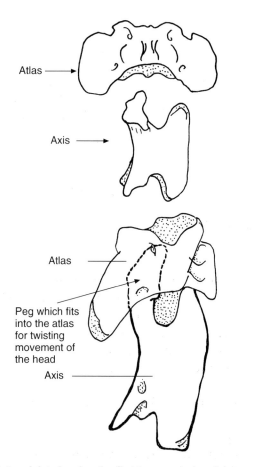

**Fig. 3.38** Pivot or rotatory joint showing the first two cervical vertebrae.

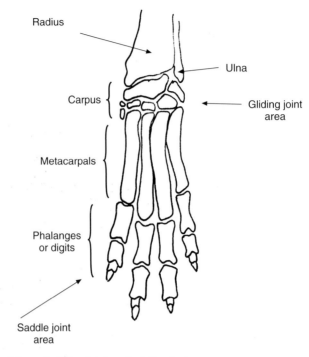

**Fig. 3.39** Saddle and gliding joints – foot (foreleg).

# Reproductive system

Reproduction refers to the formation of more individuals, from one parent (asexually) or from two parents (sexually).

Different species have evolved different processes but in all species, from plants to mammals, reproduction is closely associated with protection against adverse conditions and survival over unfavourable periods.

Mammal reproduction is by a sexual process and the male and female reproductive anatomy is very similar (Figs 3.40 and 3.41).

## *The reproductive process*

Every cell in every organism contains a set of instructions (genetic material) in chemical form for building the whole of the new organism. The set of instructions are called *chromosomes* and are situated in the nucleus of each cell. Reproduction is via special cells, produced only by the reproductive organs. Mammals have the most advanced reproductive systems in the animal kingdom. Not only do they have internal fertilisation, they have internal development as well.

Internal development has the advantage that the female mammal does not have to remain in one place, as birds do when incubating their eggs, but can lead a reasonably normal life during pregnancy. This also assists in the survival of a species.

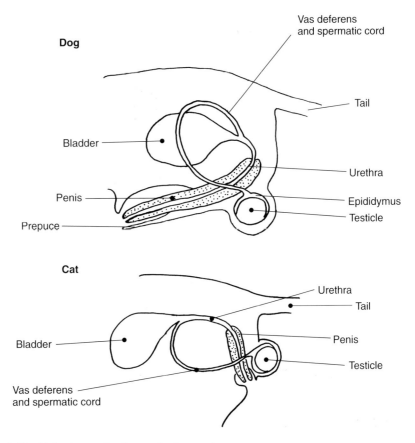

**Fig. 3.40**   Male dog and cat reproductive anatomy.

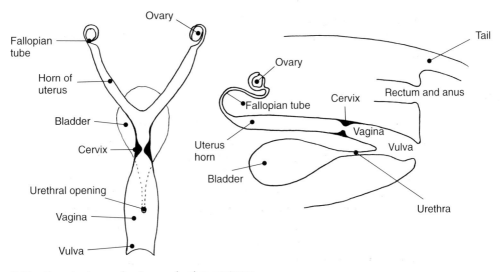

**Fig. 3.41**   Female dog and cat reproductive anatomy.

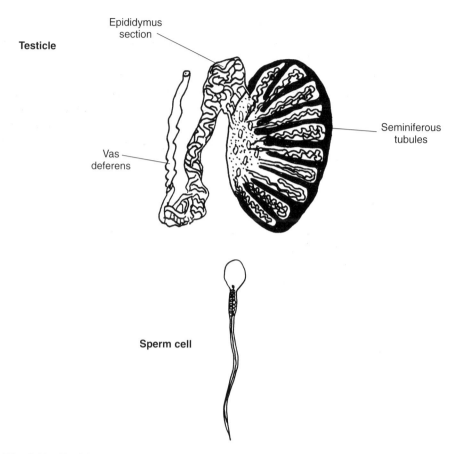

**Fig. 3.43**   Testicle and sperm cell.

### *Oestrus*

This is the period of sexual receptivity and, depending on species, may last from one to several days. During the rest of the oestrus cycle, the female does not accept the male's advances or allow mating. The cycle is made up of four or five stages, depending on the species and whether the animal is *polyoestrus* (cycles repeatedly like the cat, rat or Hamster) or is *monoestrus* (cycles only once during the breeding season, like the dog).

#### *The stages of oestrus*

- *Anoestrus* – the end of the breeding season, with no activity on the part of the reproductive organs.
- *Pro-oestrus* – just before oestrus, follicle-stimulating hormone secretion causes the follicles to develop in the ovary. FSH stimulates the ovary to release increased amounts of oestrogen, causing changes to the reproductive tract and preparing for pregnancy.

- *Oestrus* – will accept a male. Release of the ova (ovulation) occurs. FSH levels decrease and luteinizing hormone increases, causing the ripened Graafian follicles to rupture, releasing the ova.
- *Metoestrus* – the period in which hormone activity fades and tissues are less active. If the ovum has been fertilised, the corpus luteum forms and produces progesterone, which is responsible for maintaining pregnancy. Oestrogen secretions decrease. If pregnancy does not occur, the corpus luteum decreases in size, reducing the production of progesterone. This is followed by anoestrus and the cycle starts once more.

### Signs of heat

- Calling, can be very vocal, especially in cats
- More affectionate
- Restless
- Seeking the male animal
- Rolling and appearing submissive

# Chapter 4
# Basic Genetics

## Introduction

### Mendel's first law

Mendelian inheritance is the basis of all genetic practice, but it has limitations, in explaining the small differences that occur in a range of offspring of similar and related matings. Mendel was an Austrian abbot who studied and researched this variation in offspring. He used as his experimental model pea plants, which set out the basis of modern genetics.

The cells of each individual, what ever the species, are unique to that individual. All the cells of that body will contain the same set of instructions, since all were produced from the same fertilised egg. These instructions assist cells to develop as the united body and will work together for the life and health of that body.

### Chromosomes and genes

The nucleus of all cells contains the threads of DNA. DNA acts as a chemical building blueprint which is stored in each nucleus in coded form. As a result of this blueprint, the DNA can produce exact copies of itself and instructions can be passed on to new cells that form in the body.

DNA is stored in the nucleus of a cell in structures called *chromosomes*. The number of chromosomes in each species of animal will be different and specific to that species. Chromosomes are always found in pairs.

Genes are a unit of heredity most simply defined as a specific segment of DNA. Many characteristics are determined by a single gene. Genes control all aspects of the body, whether it is the coat, hair or eye colour, rate of bone growth or the ability of the blood to clot. Unfortunately, genes are responsible for many diseases and disorders as well, which are called *inherited factors*.

Each gene has its own allocated place on a particular chromosome, called the *gene locus*. Genes that occupy the same gene locus are called *alleles* or *allelomorphs*.

**Genetic terms**

- *Dominant* – masks or suppresses the presence of a recessive gene. In order for a dominant gene (B) to be expressed, the genotype is either Bb or BB.
- *Recessive* – only produces characteristics if interited from both parents. In order for a recessive gene (b) to be expressed, the genotype must be bb.
- *Homozygous* – contains the same alleles of a gene, like BB or bb.
- *Heterozygous* – if the alleles are different, like B or b.
- *Phenotype* – the appearance of an organism; for example, coat colour is black or silver.
- *Genotype* – is the actual genetic make-up.
- *Masked genes* – known as *epistasis* or masking; this happens when some genes have an overwhelming effect on others, swamping the normally occurring characteristics of the overwhelmed gene.
- *Mimic genes* – occur when distinctly different genes produce similar bodily effects; for example, the rex gene in cats. These two breeds look similar but genetically are quite different.
- *Rogue genes* – these produce bad or life-threatening effects on the body, including:
  (a)   extra toes
  (b)   lack of any hair/coat
  (c)   undescended testicles
  (d)   eyesight defects, like the Siamese gene
  (e)   deafness, as in white gene animals.

## Cell division

There are two methods of cell division, depending on the cells involved.

### Mitosis

Refers to normal body cell division (skin, muscle, etc.). Before a cell divides, copies of each chromosome form alongside the originals and then separate from the originals. As a cell divides, a full set of chromosomes collect at each end to form part of the two new cell nuclei. This method ensures that full chemical instructions are passed on to the new cells.

### Meiosis

Refers to the division of cells involved in reproduction of a new individual only. Its purpose is to form sex cells (*gametes*). The result of meiosis is that each sperm and each egg contains one member of each pair of chromosomes. Containing exactly one half of the usual diploid number of chromosomes, gametes are said to be *haploid*. The union of a sperm with an egg at

## Homoeostasis

Homoeostasis is the state of equilibrium in the body with respect to various functions and the chemical composition of fluids and tissues. The word 'homoeostasis' means 'staying the same'. Some of the factors which must be kept the same are:

- Chemical constituents like glucose and electrolytes (salts)
- Osmotic pressure and the movement of fluid (water) and substances carried by this water
- Levels of the waste gas carbon dioxide
- Body temperature

Other products must be eliminated from the body because of their harmful effect. The most important of these are the nitrogenous waste products arising from protein metabolism and toxic substances released by micro-organisms that live in the body.

### *Internal environment*

This refers to the immediate surroundings of the cells. The cells are surrounded by tiny channels and spaces filled with fluid and the fluid can be identified by the following names:

- Intercellular (between)
- Extracellular interstitial
- Tissue fluid

The cells are provided with a medium in which they live and this represents the organism's internal environment, which must be kept constant if the cells are to continue their vital functions. This fluid will return to the bloodstream eventually, either by osmotic pressure or via the lymph.

Other examples of homoeostasic mechanisms in the body include the following:

- The regulation of sugar levels in the bloodstream. It may be broken down and used as energy at the cellular level, stored in the liver as glycogen, converted to fat for storage or released into the bloodstream to top up the circulating levels.
- The above cannot be achieved without the various hormone chemical messengers provided by the organs of the endocrine system.
- The nervous system receives information from the body about all products and whether they are at the correct levels. If not, it sends a message to the organs concerned to rectify the situation.

In order to control homoeostasis, the body has feedback mechanisms. The sense organs feed back information to the brain and from here messages are sent to the relevant system or tissue for a response. The results of this response are then fed back to the brain, which decides on any subsequent action.

There is an important difference between homoeostatic feedback and a voluntary or conscious control action by the body. In homoeostasis, feedback is largely an unconscious activity – the animal is unaware that it is taking place.

Homoeostasis is most highly developed in mammals and birds, probably as a result of their evolution. They are able to maintain a constant body temperature despite environmental temperature change. This is greatly assisted by feathers and fur for insulation.

# Section 2
# Animal Health and Husbandry

# Chapter 6
# Animal Welfare

## Welfare status

Welfare has many different aspects. There is no simple scale of expression and the problems are many and diverse in their nature. One method of expressing this diversity is known as 'The Five Freedoms', which particularly relate to UK farm animal welfare and suggest that the following are essential for quality of life:

- Freedom from hunger and thirst
- Freedom to express normal behaviour
- Freedom from discomfort
- Freedom from pain, injury and disease
- Freedom from fear or distress

The above was initially set out to provide a useful framework for farm animal welfare and guidance but it is also a suggested framework for companion animals.

---

**Welfare terms**

*Animal welfare* – refers to an animal's:

- quality of life
- conditions
- treatment

It is a concept which involves values as well as information. These values consider the ways in which humans continue to use animals and whether or not this 'use' constitutes animal abuse.

*Animal rights* – refers to the total abolition of animal use in industries, recreation and other practices, as cruel, unethical and outdated.

*Conservation* – refers to the consideration of the needs of one species, above another, of animals in the wild; the promotion of human understanding and education of animal habitats, affinity with certain species and the direct effect human activity can have on their welfare and survival.

---

## Legislation

This covers both laws and regulations specific to the welfare of an animal or animal collection. These are combined with the professional working standards set by carers of animals.

Laws are guidelines and are changing all the time. It is therefore the responsibility of all animal carers to:

- Maintain a practical working knowledge of the law relating to animals
- Always work within that law

Legislation in the UK refers to both Acts of Parliament and Regulations.

- *Laws* (statutes) – are created by Parliament. Presented as draft legislation in the form of a bill, they are debated in the House of Commons and the House of Lords initially. It is then considered by specifically formed parliamentary committee, before finally receiving the Queen's signature to become law and being placed in the Statute book as an Act of Parliament.
- *Regulations* (orders) – these detail the technical implications of laws. The relevant government minister adds regulations to the legislation. This information is a supplement to existing law and must have the approval of Parliament.

Welfare codes must also have parliamentary approval. Failure to comply with the provisions of a code is not in itself an offence but could be used in evidence if prosecuted.

In addition to the above, we must abide by standards set by the European Union (EU) which have been incorporated into and take precedence over UK law.

Animal welfare legislation aims to:

- Balance concern for ethics and morality
- Balance financial and practical working considerations
- Ensure public health and safety
- State housing and transport requirements
- Maintain animal health
- Control licensing

Areas of the law relating to animal concerns in the UK are:

(1) Protection of the public laws
(2) Welfare laws to cover:
   - keeping of animals for commercial reasons
   - cruelty laws

(3)   Animal collection laws
(4)   Welfare of wild animals laws

## Protection of the public laws

- Animal Health Act 1981
- Dangerous Dogs Acts 1991, 1997
- Guard Dogs Act 1975
- Animals Act 1971
- Dogs Fouling of Land Act 1996

### Animal Health Act 1981 and quarantine regulations

This Act gives government ministers powers to make orders to control introduction and spread of zoonotic disease and assist in the eradication of diseases carried by animals in the UK. The orders and regulations covered include the following:

- The Rabies (Control) Order 1974, now incorporated into the Animal Health Act
- Quarantine for imports and exports
- Points of entry to Britain
- Transport method and conditions
- Seizure of animals and their disposal (dogs and wildlife)
- Disinfection of places and vehicles

The Kennedy Advisory Group was appointed to look at existing regulations and make recommendations for replacing quarantine. The government intends to introduce the Kennedy-style arrangements by April 2001. The new scheme proposes to allow dogs and cats coming from EU countries, certain other European countries and rabies-free islands to enter the UK without having to undergo quarantine provided they can be shown to meet the necessary criteria regarding vaccination and identification. This would not apply to dogs and cats entering Britain from the USA and Canada.

Requirements:

- Microchipped with electronic chip
- Vaccinated against rabies using an inactivated vaccine
- Treated for exotic diseases not in the UK
- Blood tested at an approved laboratory
- Has an official health certificate

Enforcing the new system:

- Pre-entry checks carried out by train operators, ferry companies and airlines
- Random spot checks on animals arriving in the UK by MAFF and official carriers

### Dangerous Dogs Acts 1991, 1997

After an increase in the number of attacks on people by dogs in the 1980s and 1990s, some fatal, the government introduced laws making it more difficult to own and import into the UK the following breeds of dog:

- American pit bull terrier
- Japanese tossa
- Dogo Argentino
- Fila Braziliera

The Act states that the rules for ownership of a dangerous named breed of dog are as follows:

- Notifying the police of ownership.
- Obtaining a certificate of exemption from the police, which is issued when the dog has been neutered and identified with a microchip or other permanent method.
- The dog is covered by third party liability insurance.
- In public places, the dog is always muzzled and on a lead.
- In the company of a person over 16 years of age.
- It is an offence to sell, exchange or abandon the dog.
- It is an offence to breed from these dogs.

Any dog dangerously out of control and a risk to the general public comes under the remit of this Act. The person in charge of a dog that has inflicted injury could be prosecuted and face an unlimited fine or prison sentence.

### Guard Dogs Act 1975

This Act ensures the safe use and control of dogs which guard property or sites and in a manner which does not put the general public at risk. A notice must be on display to inform the public that a dog is in use and the dog must only be off the lead if accompanied by a handler.

### Animals Act 1971

This Act covers liability for damage that has been caused by animals, including damage, death and injury caused to people, property and livestock. The owner of a dangerous animal must take precautions to ensure it has no opportunity to inflict damage as stated by this law. If a dog kills or harms farm animals, farmers are entitled to protect the stock in their care. If, for example, a dog is found injuring sheep the farmer may kill the dog but must report the incident to the police.

### Dog Fouling of Land Act 1996

Local authorities and councils use this Act to prevent dogs fouling where there is public access to property or pavements but allowing exemption of guide dogs for the blind.

## Welfare laws

Those keeping animals for commercial reasons:

* Animal Boarding Establishment Act 1963
* Breeding of Dogs Act 1973
* Pet Animals Acts 1951, 1983

Cruelty laws:

* Protection of Animals Acts 1911, 1988
* Protection of Animals (Anaesthetics) Acts 1954, 1982
* Veterinary Surgeons Act 1966

### Animal Boarding Establishment Act 1963

The main provision of this Act is that boarding kennels or catteries must be licensed by their local authority in order to trade. The following conditions apply:

* Records kept of animal arrivals and departures and details of owners
* Provision of suitable accommodation
* Adequate and appropriate supplies of food and water
* Exercise facilities available
* Animals protected from disease and risk of fire

In order to ensure that the conditions of the licence are met, the local authority can at any time instruct inspection by an authorised officer or veterinary surgeon. Licences are renewed annually.

### Breeding of Dogs Acts 1963, 1991

The law altered in 1991, allowing authorised officers or veterinary surgeons to enter premises with a warrant if they suspect an offence under the 1963 Act has been committed. The term 'breeding establishment' refers to any premises where more than two bitches are kept for the purpose of breeding animals for selling.

The 1963 Act prohibits:

- Obstruction of inspection by authorised personnel
- Breeding dogs for sale without a licence from the local authority
- If disqualified under other Acts of Parliament, holding a licence for breeding of dogs

*Pet Animals Acts 1951, 1983*

This Act was introduced at the end of World War II in response to the worrying number of animals being sold in street markets and pet shops with no restrictions or controls for conditions or care. The Act prohibits the keeping of a pet shop without a licence. A licence is granted after inspection of premises by an approved veterinary surgeon authorised by the local authority. The Act was amended in 1983, making it illegal to sell pets in public places. A licence is granted if the following conditions are met:

- Proper care
- Suitable accommodation
- Housed in the correct conditions with reference to heating, lighting, etc.
- Provided with appropriate food
- Observed and checked at suitable intervals during the day
- Sold only after weaning and a suitable age has been reached
- Prevention of spread of disease
- Emergency and fire precautions for the premises are in place and functional

*Protection of Animals Acts 1911, 1988*

This series of Acts forms the main statutory control on cruelty to animals by humans. These Acts are used when bringing prosecutions related to animal welfare cases. The Act makes it an offence to cause unnecessary suffering to any domestic or captive animal either deliberately or by omission (neglect). The Act lists offences such as:

- Inflicting physical cruelty by beating, kicking, etc.
- Inflicting mental cruelty by teasing or terrifying
- Causing unnecessary suffering during transportation by failing to provide food or water at appropriate intervals
- Performing surgery or operations without an anaesthetic
- Poisoning without reason

*Protection of Animals (Anaesthetics) Acts 1954, 1982*

It is illegal for any operation to be conducted on an animal that will cause pain unless under anaesthetic (local or general). There are, however, several exceptions to this Act:

- Does not apply to birds, fish or reptiles
- In emergency first aid situations
- Under permitted Home Office-licensed procedures
- Minor painless operations carried out by a veterinary surgeon or a listed veterinary nurse

*Veterinary Surgeons Act 1966*

This Act prohibits anyone other than a veterinary surgeon or listed veterinary nurse registered with the Royal College of Veterinary Surgeons from carrying out treatment or operations on animals. The exceptions to this are:

- Minor treatments given by owner, household member or employee of the owner
- Castration or tail docking of lambs provided they are under a stated age
- Emergency first aid to maintain life

## Animal collection laws

- Welfare of Animals during Transport 1973, 1994 (Amendment) Order 1995
- Abandonment of Animals Act 1960
- Dangerous Wild Animals Act 1976
- Performing Animals (Regulation) Act 1925
- Zoo Licensing Act 1981

*Welfare of Animals during Transport 1973, 1994 (Amendment) Order 1995*

This order is designed to protect all animals during transport by road, rail, sea and air. From 1997, a standard set of regulations on journey times, hauliers' journey plans and routes covering EU countries amended the original order. The regulations cover:

- Loading and unloading of animals
- Housing and containers for transit
- Access to food and water
- Specified number of animals contained together for transit

*Abandonment of Animals Act 1960*

This Act applies to the abandonment of an animal in circumstances likely to cause it unnecessary suffering. This would apply to an owner or person in control of a companion animal who has abandoned it either completely or for only a temporary period of time.

*Dangerous Wild Animals Act 1976*

This Act became necessary when, in the 1960s and 1970s, the public started to keep animals more frequently associated with zoos and safari parks – animals such as leopards, lions, various types of monkey and many other dangerous wild animals. Animals were often kept in poor conditions and insecure housing, causing concern both for their welfare and for people living nearby.

Public demand led to legislation and strict control and inspection by authorised veterinary surgeons who may inspect premises in which these animals are kept. If the inspection is approved, a licence is issued by the local authority.

The Secretary of State has the power to change the list of animals at any time and any animal on the list is classified as a 'dangerous wild animal'. The Act states that anyone keeping these listed animals must:

- Pay a fee to the local authority for the issue of the licence
- Take out liability insurance
- Provide suitable accommodation
- Be over 18 years of age

*Performing Animals (Regulation) Act 1925*

A Select Committee of the House of Lords introduced this Act following public concern over the treatment of animals in circuses. As a result, the local authority must be informed of anyone who trains animals for exhibition to the public or exhibits a performing animal to the public, even if it is free of charge, and any such person must be registered to that effect.

The exceptions to this rule are when animals are trained for sporting purposes, military or police work and display.

*Zoo Licensing Act 1981*

The term 'zoo' refers to the exhibiting of wild animals to the public, for educational purposes. It applies to animal collections which are open to the public for seven days or more in any year.

This Act was passed after the dramatic increase of zoos and wildlife/safari parks in the 1960s. It is intended to protect the zoo animals and the general public by ensuring that standards of care, the welfare of the animals and the safety of the public are in place.

The zoo must obtain a licence from the local authority, which is renewed initially after four years and then every six years.

### The welfare of wild animals laws

- The Wildlife and Countryside Acts 1981, 1985
- Convention of International Trade in Endangered Species of Wild Flora and Fauna (CITES) 1973

#### The Wildlife and Countryside Acts 1981, 1985

These Acts replace several existing laws and regulations and cover the protection and conservation of wild animals and their habitats. Land, sea and airborne species of wild animals are protected. The minister can add or remove species on this list, which may not legally be injured, killed or taken from the wild.

The Act protects habitat from humans and species in captivity which, if released into the wild, would seriously affect many other species.

Within the Act, licences can be granted which exempt the holder from the above provisions:

- Relating to the protection of farming or forestry interests
- Relating to the conservation, reintroducing, photographing and identification of wildlife

#### Convention on international trade in endangered species of wild flora and fauna (CITES) 1973

This international agreement helps to protect the world's endangered species by controlling their export and import on a worldwide scale. Animals in this category are classed in two ways:

- Those that are threatened with extinction
- Those likely to become so threatened

## Statutory organisations

### Royal Society for the Prevention of Cruelty to Animals Act 1932 (RSPCA)

The Society was founded in 1824 by the Reverend Arthur Broome. Its aim is to promote kindness and prevent cruelty to animals. The Act of 1932 empowers the RSPCA to act in certain situations concerning the welfare of animals.

The RSPCA:

- Operates throughout England and Wales, maintaining animal homes and clinics
- Prosecutes in cases of cruelty
- Lobbies on animal welfare issues throughout Europe
- Conducts discreet surveillance of activities, such as livestock transportation abroad
- Funds research into animal welfare
- Maintains links with affiliated organisations in the European community

### People's Dispensary for Sick Animals Act 1949 (PDSA)

Founded in 1917 by Maria Dickin, the initial aim of the PDSA was to help sick and injured animals in the east end of London. It provides free veterinary treatment to sick and injured animals when owners are unable to afford treatment. It is not involved with neutering or vaccinations. It has treatment centres and hospitals all over the country as well as the Pet Aid scheme involving general practices in some counties.

### Royal College of Veterinary Surgeons, Veterinary Surgeons Act 1981

The college was established to teach, train and examine people who wished to become registered as a veterinary surgeon. In order to remain on the RCVS register, members pay an annual fee. The Act established a council responsible for regulating its membership and ensuring unqualified people did not use the title of veterinary surgeon, treat or operate on animals.

# Chapter 7
# Basic Health Care

Basic health care refers to the daily, weekly, monthly and lifelong observations by the owner, carer or handler. Health care is the regular and routine examination of an animal to identify any abnormalities and keep it in the best of health. This could refer to checking a dog's ears weekly for signs of wax or the length of tooth check on a pet rabbit.

Early recognition of signs of ill health is important to diagnosis and treatment. Owners and carers know what is normal for each animal in their care.

Signs of health include:

- Lack of discharge from eyes and ears
- Eyes clear and bright
- Good coat/feather condition
- Correct weight
- Alert and responds to stimuli
- Eats and drinks normal quantities
- Urinates and defecates without difficulty
- Enjoys exercise

Signs of ill health include:

- Vomiting and/or diarrhoea
- Breathing difficulties
- Discharges from eyes, ears, nose, prepuce or vulva
- Scratching and hair/feather loss
- Unwilling to exercise
- Not responding to stimuli
- Pain on movement

It is important that, from an early age, the animal is used to handling. This means that when there is a problem and the animal is taken to the veterinary surgeon for examination, it is not further distressed. Examining feet and ears on, for example, a puppy or kitten from an early age will mean they are much more tolerant and no one gets bitten or scratched.

- Remove urine-soiled bedding.
- Disinfect housing.

### *Weekly hygiene*

- Wash bedding.
- Wash nylon harness or collars.
- Groom (Fig. 7.3).
- Disinfect grooming equipment.

## Exercise

Each animal has specific exercise needs. In the case of dogs, many potential owners will partly base their decision to buy a particular breed on its energy levels and exercise requirements.

A breed such as a border collie has a high requirement whereas a breed like the pug has a much lower one. Breed books clearly state requirements for exercise, temperament and suitability for potential owners. Life stages and lifespan will suggest the exercise needs.

Plenty of exercise is necessary for breeds used in the areas of:

- Working
- Racing
- Performance
- Agility
- Field trials

Less exercise is required for:

- Elderly animals
- Short-nosed breeds (brachycephalic)
- Some small breeds
- Those with joint disease
- Those with breathing and heart conditions

Cats tend to 'self exercise' but can be trained to walk on a lead. Small pets will exercise if they have enhanced living areas with obstacles for climbing, toys and run areas, plus handling time.

## Tender loving care

An important aspect of health care is time spent in the company of the animal. Owners, carers and handlers can use this time to run health status checks. Dogs and cats should be companion animals. Dogs particularly are pack animals and respond badly to isolation.

Signs of isolation response include:

- Temperament change
- Destruction of housing
- Being aggressive or withdrawn
- Fear

The above list could perfectly describe the normal behaviour of an individual. The only way to know is to recognise what is normal for each individual, whatever the species.

## Vaccination

This is a means of protecting an animal against a potentially lethal disease. Vaccines temporarily stimulate the immune system of the body. The period of protection will vary depending on the species involved, the vaccine type and the individual receiving the vaccine. It ranges in most cases from six months to one year, at which point the animal must receive a booster vaccination to protect it further.

# Chapter 8
# Disease Transmission and Control

Disease is spread from one animal to another by various methods. Microbes leave the body in or on:

- Oral, nasal and eye discharges, e.g. rabies via the saliva, feline respiratory diseases and distemper via eye and nose discharge
- Urine, e.g. causing leptospirosis and hepatitis
- Vomit, e.g. causing parvo in dogs
- Blood, e.g. transmitted by fleas to another animal
- Skin surface, e.g. surface bacteria and fungi like ringworm
- Milk from mother to offspring passing worms and some viruses

The microbes are passed on from one animal to another, sometimes by a carrier animal. These animals do not show clinical signs of disease but are:

- Individuals that have had the disease and recovered, called *convalescent carriers*
- Individuals that never show clinical signs of the disease and are called *healthy carriers*

Both types will shed the disease-carrying microbe into the environment, putting other animals at risk. The microbe is passed from one animal to another by:

- *Direct contact* – parts of the bodies of two animals come into contact, e.g. nose to nose or nose to anus
- *Indirect contact* – the contact is on an inanimate object, e.g. bedding, water bowl or lamp post
- *Aerosol transmission* – through the air, in the form of droplets from sneezing, coughing or using air currents
- *Contaminated food or water* – contaminated by urine and faeces of passing rodents or others (due to incorrect storage of dried foods)
- *Carrier animals* – shedding microbes in discharges, urine or faeces yet unaffected themselves, e.g. canine hepatitis

## Incubation of the disease

Incubation refers to the time between the animal receiving the microbe and showing clinical signs of disease. It will depend on:

- *Quantity of microbes received* – if received via the respiratory and/or digestive tracts, secretions here and movement of particles will prevent microbes establishing, unless the animal is susceptible.
- *Immune status of the animal* – it may fail to mount an adequate immune response, allowing the microbes to move on to other target tissues and establish themselves.
- *General health* – if not good, then the animal is susceptible.
- *Age* – the immune response of the body is reduced with age.

## Entry into a new host

### Eating

- Infected food/water
- Contact with contaminated food/water bowls
- Eating faeces (*coprophagia*)
- Eating the disease carrier, e.g. flea, while grooming itself

### Inhalation

- Breathing in airborne microbes, or by sniffing contaminated surface

### Through the skin

- Wound
- Scratch
- Insect bite
- Subsurface mite like sarcoptes

### Via damaged mucous membranes

- Mouth
- Nose
- Eye

## Infection

If the micro-organism has entered the host animal and overcome its resistance, infection may ensue. Some infections are confined to a restricted area, e.g.

abscesses; others are called *systemic* because they spread through the whole body via the bloodstream.

---

**Infection terms**

- *Subclinical infection* – has no clinical signs
- *Bacteraemia* – bacteria are present in the bloodstream
- *Pyaemia* – bacteria and white blood cells forming pus are in the blood
- *Septicaemia* – bacteria multiply in the bloodstream

---

## Resistance to infection

Individual resistance will depend on:

- Age
- Nutritional state (too thin or overweight)
- Skin being intact
- Vaccination status
- Immune response and white cell activity

## Methods of disease control

- Avoid direct contact with infected animals (use of isolation).
- High levels of hygiene/disinfection in the animal's environment.
- Reduce the number of animals kept within the same air space or improve the efficiency of air movement to reduce aerosol transmission.
- Provide early and effective treatment of infected animals to prevent others becoming infected.
- Control parasites to prevent passing of disease from one animal to another.
- Maintain vaccination status.

# Chapter 9
# Microbiology

## Micro-organisms (microbes)

Microbiology is the study and identification of micro-organisms.

- Bacteria
- Viruses
- Fungi
- Protozoa

Micro-organisms are measured in *micrometres* or *microns*: 1 micron = 1 thousandth of a millimetre. Microbes range from large protozoa to the virus, which is the smallest. Viruses can only be seen using an electron microscope and are measured in *nanometres*: 1 nanometre = 1 millionth of a millimetre.

Microbes are described according to their nutritional requirements.

- *Autotrophs* – synthesise (create) their own food
- *Heterotrophs* – obtain nutrients from their environment

Microbes live throughout the environment of humans and animals and are normally present on or within the body.

---

**Microbial terms**

- *Infection* – process by which microbes become established in the host.
- *Saprophytes* – live and feed on dead organic material.
- *Symbiosis* – the association between two different species, living together.
- *Parasitic* – refers to the association between two different living organisms in which the parasite lives upon the host, taking food and shelter (host's own food or body fluids). Parasites fall into three groups:
  - (a) *pathogens* – will harm the host animal, causing disease
  - (b) *commensals* – will not harm but nor will they benefit the host
  - (c) *mutualistics* – are of benefit to the host, e.g. help break down food in the gut in some species.

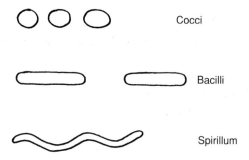

Cocci

Bacilli

Spirillum

**Fig. 9.1**   Shapes of bacteria.

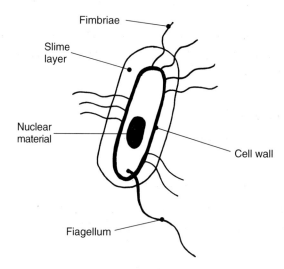

Fimbriae

Slime layer

Nuclear material

Cell wall

Fiagellum

**Fig. 9.2**   Bacterium in detail.

# Bacteria

Most range from 0.5 to 5 microns in length. They may be rod shaped (bacillus), round or spherical (cocci) or spiral shaped (Fig. 9.1).

## *Structure (Fig. 9.2)*

- *Cell wall* – for shape and protection.
- *Capsule or loose slime layer* – for sticking to surfaces, protection from its environment and preventing destruction by phagocytic white blood cells.
- *Plasma membrane* – controls the passage of substances in and out of the cell.
- *Internal cell organelles* (cytoplasm, ribosomes, etc.) – to support the life of the cell.
- *Flagellum and pili* – hair-like structures for moving the cells along.

## Reproduction of bacteria

This takes place providing the following are available:

- Supply of nutrients
- Correct temperature
- Correct pH and oxygen levels

Not all bacteria require oxygen.

- *Aerobic bacteria* – grow in the presence of free oxygen
- *Anaerobic bacteria* – only grow in the absence of free oxygen

Bacteria reproduce by growth and then division of the cell. Most reproduce by an asexual method called *binary fission*. For many bacteria, division takes 15–20 minutes.

### Binary fission

One cell divides into two cells (Fig. 9.3).

### Conjugation or bacterial mating

Sexual reproduction refers to the passing of genetic material and information from a bacterial donor to a recipient bacterium. It is passed through a short tube,

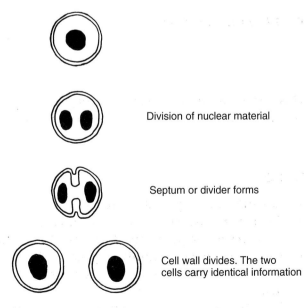

Division of nuclear material

Septum or divider forms

Cell wall divides. The two cells carry identical information

**Fig. 9.3**   Binary fission.

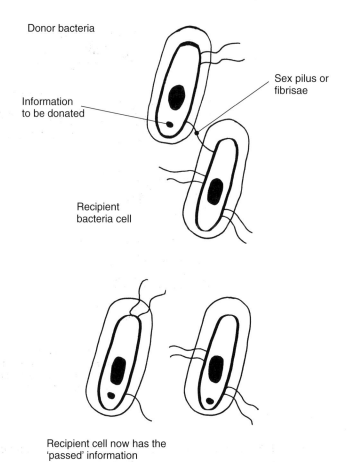

Donor bacteria

Sex pilus or
fibrisae

Information
to be donated

Recipient
bacteria cell

Recipient cell now has the
'passed' information

**Fig. 9.4**  Conjugation or bacterial mating.

the *sex pilus* (Fig. 9.4). This method passes part of the donor cell chromosome and extra genes, e.g. genes carrying antibiotic resistance factor, to another bacterium.

Some bacteria produce a dormant spore form (*endospore*). The production of spores is similar to binary fission but the septum or divider is nearer one end of the cell and grows to surround the genetic information. This creates a spore, the

---

**Bacterial terms**

- *Endotoxins* – toxins produced within the bacteria, only released into the host animal when the bacteria die. The toxins can cause signs of shock or fever and can be lethal.
- *Exotoxins* – toxins secreted by the living bacteria which can also be harmful to the host animal's body.

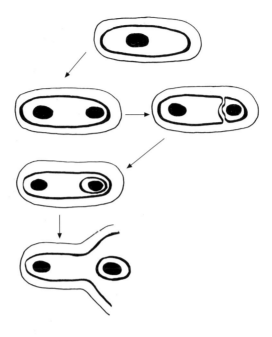

Cell finally ruptures to
release spore which will remain
in this form, protected, until its
environment improves

**Fig. 9.5**   Spore formation.

genetic information being contained within a protective coat or covering. This
spore will form when conditions for life are not favourable, e.g. nutrients are not
available. Once the spore forms, the original cell breaks down or *lyses*, releasing
the spore into the environment to await improved conditions (Fig. 9.5). This is
not a form of reproduction but a means of survival.

## Viruses

Viruses are the smallest of the microbes (Fig. 9.6). They are always parasitic and
reproduce by replicating themselves. This process happens after the viral DNA
or RNA (genetic information) has entered a host animal's body cell. This strand
of material takes over control of the host cell's metabolism and directs it to manufacture replicas of the viral material. When enough replicas have been produced,
the virus will instruct the host cell to rupture, releasing the new viruses which go
on to use other host cells for the purpose of replicating.

    The virus is not a cell. In structure, it is a protein coat around a DNA or RNA
strand. Some viruses are also surrounded by a membrane known as an *envelope*
which may have structures like spikes on its surface for attaching to the host cell
before entry.

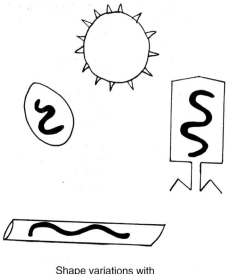

Shape variations with
DNA strand and protein coat
for protection

**Fig. 9.6**   Examples of virus shapes.

In many cases, the cycle of viral infection causes no apparent harm to the host. Disease occurs when the host is harmed by the infection which occurs when quantities of host cells have been destroyed.

## Fungi

These are non-chlorophyll bearing plants, often called *hyphae* and divided into:

- *Moulds* – multicellular
- *Yeasts* – unicellular

They do not have the ability to create their own food and so must exist as parasites or saprophytes. Distribution is by spores (Fig. 9.7).

Reproduction is sexual (hyphae from different strains unite into a survival spore form, awaiting favourable conditions) and there is also an asexual method (distribution of spores). Examples of diseases caused by fungi are ringworm and dermatophytes.

## Protozoa

These are single-celled animals and range in size from microscopic to just visible to the naked eye. They have a cell membrane and have organelles for movement (flagella and cilia) (Fig. 9.8). Reproduction is asexual by binary fission.

Diseases produced by different microbes.

| Microbe | Dog | Cat |
|---|---|---|
| Protozoa | Coccidiosis<br>Toxoplasmosis | Coccidiosis<br>Toxoplasmosis |
| Fungi | Ringworm | Ringworm |
| Bacteria | Kennel cough<br>Leptospirosis | |
| Virus | Distemper<br>Infectious hepatitis<br>Parvovirus<br>Rabies | Panleucopenia<br>Respiratory disease<br>Infectious peritonitis<br>Leukaemia<br>Immunodeficiency<br>Rabies |

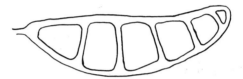

Spindle-shaped cells which make
up the spore, as seen in
*Microsporum canis* ringworm

**Fig. 9.7**  Fungal spore.

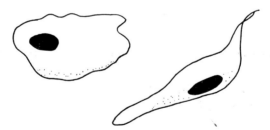

**Fig. 9.8**  Protozoa forms.

Nutrition is *holozoic* (capture and assimilation of organic material in their environment). Protozoa are capable of pursuing prey by following a chemical trail or they can be stimulated by movement, particularly in water.

Protozoa will form a *cyst* at some point in their life cycle. This is the form which passes from host to host and allows temporary survival outside the host.

Diseases caused by protozoa include toxoplasmosis and coccidiosis.

# Chapter 10
# Diseases of the Dog and Cat

## Diseases of dogs

The infectious canine diseases for which there is a vaccine include:

- Canine distemper
- Canine viral hepatitis
- Canine leptospirosis
- Canine parvovirus
- Canine infectious tracheobronchitis (kennel cough syndrome)
- Rabies

### Canine distemper

The virus causing distemper attacks the following body systems:

- Central nervous system
- Respiratory system
- Gastrointestinal system
- Skin

The disease is caused by a paramyxovirus that is closely related to the measles virus of humans. The virus is inactivated by light, heat and most disinfectants.

Distemper is commonly seen in puppies of 4–5 months when no longer covered by maternal immunity. It has a seasonal occurrence in autumn and winter, due in part to the ability of the virus to survive in cold weather.

Routes of infection into a new host animal are:

- Respiratory tract due to aerosol (airborne) exposure
- Mouth and eye mucous membranes

During the incubation period of 3–10 days, the virus replicates and travels via the lymphatic system to the lymph nodes, spleen, thymus and bone marrow. When in the lymph nodes, body temperature rises to between 39 and 40°C for 2–4 days.

About half of all puppies infected are capable of mounting an adequate response and produce antibodies to clear the infection at this point. If the virus continues, it replicates in the epithelium, organs and central nervous system. This allows secondary infection to occur.

Clinical signs include:

- Lack of appetite (*anorexia*)
- Nasal and eye discharge
- Coughing
- Diarrhoea and vomiting
- Hardening of the footpads
- Inco-ordination
- Paralysis
- Epileptic-type fits

If the puppy survives the respiratory or gastrointestinal stage of the disease, the neurological signs develop up to four weeks later. Older dogs tend to present with just the neurological signs. This is usually fatal; occasionally the dog will survive but there will be lasting central nervous system damage.

Vaccination gives good protection but is not lifelong, so booster vaccinations are essential.

### Canine infectious tracheobronchitis (kennel cough syndrome)

The micro-organisms causing kennel cough syndrome include:

- *Bordetella bronchiseptica*
- Canine adenovirus type 2 (CAV2)
- Canine parainfluenza virus (CPIV)
- Canine distemper virus (CDV)

This syndrome is a complex disease linked to a number of viruses. However, the major cause is thought to be the bacteria *Bordetella bronchiseptica*. Clinically the syndrome presents as tracheitis, which is usually self-limiting but which may also develop into bronchitis or pneumonia.

*Bordetella bronchiseptica*, CAV2 and CPIV are very contagious and commonly present when dogs are housed together, as they infect the respiratory tracts in dogs of any age. They cause nasal and tracheal inflammation lasting 5–14 days and then normally resolve, the dog making a good recovery. At this time the dog sheds the organisms in the respiratory secretions.

Clinical signs include:

- Cough
- Sneezing and nasal discharge
- Depressed but still eating
- Retching after coughing

Transmission from dog to dog can be minimised by isolation of the affected animal and by improving the kennel ventilation and disinfection routines. All dogs that are going into a boarding establishment should have been vaccinated with a mixed vaccine that includes CAV2 and CPIV.

## Canine parvovirus

Canine parvovirus is closely related to the feline panleucopenia virus. The virus is very resistant to inactivation by most disinfectants except bleach and formalin-based chemicals and can survive for months in the environment. The virus locates in lymphatic tissues and the intestinal epithelium lining. It is found in vast numbers in the faeces and vomit of infected animals and causes myocarditis and mild to severe haemorrhagic enteritis.

The route of infection is by faecal or oral contact. Damage to the bone marrow results in lack of white cells and the infection spreads from lymph cells in the gut tissues. The incubation period is 5–10 days.

Clinical signs include:

- Being dull and depressed
- Anorexia
- High temperature (up to 41°C)
- Vomiting bloodstained gastric juice
- Bloodstained diarrhoea 24 hours later
- Becomes rapidly dehydrated

Vaccination as a puppy should be followed by annual boosters for protection.

## Canine viral hepatitis

Caused by the canine adenovirus type 1 (CAV1). Transmission is through oral and nasal passages after exposure to infected materials. The virus is resistant and survives outside the body for up to 11 days in bedding, feeding bowls, urine and faeces. It can resist freezing, ultraviolet light and most disinfectants but is destroyed by heat. Following exposure, the virus localises in the tonsils and lymph nodes where primary replication occurs. The virus travels in the lymph and gains access to the bloodstream. It is attracted to the cells of the liver and kidneys, where further replication occurs, before shedding in urine and faeces. The incubation period is 5–9 days. Recovered animals can shed the virus for several months.

Clinical signs include the following:

**Puppies**
- High temperature
- Death occurs within hours

**Older dogs**
- Survive the viraemic stage
- Bloodstained vomit and diarrhoea
- Acute abdominal pain

In some dogs 'blue eye', a clouding of the cornea of the eye, occurs up to three weeks after acute infection.

Vaccination and annual boosters are essential.

## Leptospirosis

Also known as Stuttgart disease or Weil's disease in humans, leptospirosis is caused by a filament-like bacterium, *leptospira icterohaemorrhagiae*, which is a zoonone to humans.

The strains that cause the disease in dogs are:

- *Leptospira icterohaemorrhagiae* – (primary host is the rat) attacks mainly the liver
- *Leptospira canicola* – (primary host is the dog) attacks mainly the kidney

These bacteria are easily destroyed by sunlight, disinfectants and temperature extremes.

The disease is spread by direct contact, bite wounds or ingestion of infected food or water. Rodents such as rats are frequently carriers, shedding the bacteria in urine and thus contaminating water.

Incubation is 7–21 days, with severity of the disease caused depending on the susceptibility of the host animal and the strain.

Clinical signs include:

- High temperature
- Shivering and muscle pain
- Vomiting and diarrhoea
- Dehydration
- Shock
- Jaundice (mucous membranes of mouth and eye appear yellow)

Recovered animals shed the bacteria via the urine for some time after recovery. Strict isolation must be observed. Both veterinary surgeon and doctor can provide advice and information to prevent a human carer becoming infected.

An annual booster after initial vaccination is essential.

## Rabies

Rabies is caused by a rhabdovirus. It is fragile, surviving for only a short time in the environment, and is destroyed by most disinfectants, heat and light.

Transmitted in the saliva of infected animals, the virus replicates in the muscle cells at the site of infection, then travels via the peripheral nerves to the spinal cord and the brain. Once it is located in the central nervous tissues, neurological signs are observed. The virus also then travels to the salivary glands, where it is shed to infect other mammals, both human and animal. Rabies is therefore a zoonone disease.

Incubation is from 10 days to four months, the time depending on how near to the central nervous system the virus is initially placed. There are three phases or stages to the disease symptoms. However, not all will necessarily occur in all affected animals.

(1) *Preclinical stage* – lasting 2–3 days with a raised body temperature, slow eye reflexes and signs of irritation at the site of the original injury.
(2) *Excitable stage* – lasting up to one week with the animal becoming irritable, aggressive and disorientated, having difficulty standing and epileptic-type fits.
(3) *Dumb stage* – lasting 2–4 days during which the animal becomes progressively paralysed in throat and skeletal muscles, leading to salivation, respiratory difficulties, coma and death.

In some cases the preclinical stage can last for several months during which the virus is shed in the saliva.

Diagnosis is confirmed on postmortem examination of the brain and spinal cord for signs of the virus. Vaccine is available for dogs that live in countries where rabies is endemic or for travelling to a country with rabies in the wild or domestic animal population. The vaccine is given at three months of age and boostered annually.

If bitten by a suspect animal:

- clean the wound immediately using soap or antiseptic solutions
- seek medical attention straight away

## Diseases of cats

Infectious feline diseases include:

- Rabies (see Rabies in the dog, p. 115)
- Feline leukaemia
- Feline panleucopenia or feline infectious enteritis
- Chlamydiosis or feline pneumonitis
- Feline viral respiratory disease:
    (a) feline herpesvirus
    (b) feline calicivirus

- Feline infectious anaemia
- Feline infectious peritonitis
- Feline immunodeficiency

## Feline leukaemia (FLV)

The retrovirus causing feline leukaemia affects approximately 2% of cats world-wide. It is contagious and, once symptoms appear, almost always fatal. Most cats are exposed to this virus during their life and it is most commonly found where cats are in close contact.

Evidence of the virus is obtained from testing of blood samples using the FLV ELISA test.

The effect of the virus on the host cat depends on the age of the cat when it is infected and the quantity of virus received.

- Some cats become ill and apparently recover
- Some do not become ill and develop an immunity to the disease
- Some develop the disease symptoms after incubation of weeks to several years

Young kittens are most susceptible to the virus. Most die within 2–3 years of exposure or as a result of FLV-related disease conditions, which include:

- Anaemia (lack of red blood cells)
- Lymphosarcoma (tumours of the lymph system)

Clinical signs include:

- High temperature
- Vomiting and diarrhoea
- Weight loss
- Kidney disease
- Enlargement of the spleen

The virus is shed in:

- Saliva
- Faeces
- Urine
- Milk to offspring

The virus is easily destroyed by disinfectants and cannot live long outside a host. Infection can be passed via saliva in bite/fight episodes, contact with other cats or from the mother to the kittens before or after birth via the milk.

The virus replicates in the lymph tissues initially, then moves on to other target systems containing lymph tissue, such as the intestines, causing enteritis, then on to the salivary glands, the urinary and reproductive systems, causing infertility or abortion in pregnant animals.

Control of the disease is via:

- Testing, particularly in multi-cat households
- Animals testing positive being isolated from others
- Disinfection and hygiene in cat areas
- Retesting 12 weeks after positive test to ensure true result
- Testing all new cats that join a household

After two positive tests, the safe choice is to permanently isolate or euthanase the cat. Cats are vaccinated from nine weeks of age with a second dose 2–4 weeks later followed by an annual booster. Before vaccination, all cats are tested for presence of the virus in the blood.

### Feline panleucopenia or feline infectious enteritis

Feline panleucopenia is a highly infectious disease of cats, also called:

- Feline parvovirus
- Feline distemper
- Feline infectious enteritis

The disease is caused by a parvovirus, similar to canine parvovirus. The disease can affect cats of any age but is mainly responsible for deaths in young kittens.

The virus is stable and capable of surviving in the environment for months to years and is resistant to most disinfectants. The incubation period is 2–10 days following direct contact with an infected animal or ingestion of the virus. The virus targets rapidly dividing cells and tissues of the small intestines, lymph and bone marrow. It is shed in saliva, vomit, faeces and urine.

Clinical signs include:

- Diarrhoea, often bloodstained
- Dull and listless behaviour
- Abdominal pain
- Fever and dehydration

Blood testing shows a typical reduction in white blood cells (leucopenia), particularly neutrophil white cells.

The virus can cross the placenta during pregnancy and affects the foetus by targeting the brain tissue (cerebellum), causing death or abnormal nervous system development. Kittens show balance difficulties and inco-ordination at about 2–3 weeks of age if affected. If the cat survives the first week of clinical disease, careful nursing can lead to recovery but the intestine may suffer permanent damage, seen as poor absorption of nutrients and constant diarrhoeal episodes.

Vaccination using either live or inactivated vaccine (in pregnant cats) provides good immunity with a booster every 1–2 years.

### *Chlamydiosis or feline pneumonitis*

Chlamydial infection is caused by an organism which lives within cells. Chlamydiae are therefore treated like a virus, but in appearance resemble a bacterium.

*Chlamydia cati* or *psittaci* affects the conjunctiva of the eye in cats, causing severe conjunctivitis with eye discharges, sneezing and nasal discharge. The conjunctivitis may affect one or both eyes.

Transmission is thought to be via contact with eye/nose discharges, genital tract or gastrointestinal tract secretions from carrier animals. Incubation is 3–10 days.

Clinical signs include:

- Initial watery discharge in one eye, spreading to both
- Inflamed conjunctiva
- Fever
- Rubbing eyes and signs of discomfort
- In kittens, diarrhoea

During pregnancy, chlamydia may cause abortion or stillbirth.

Chlamydiosis may last for 2–3 weeks or longer, especially as a part of the feline viral respiratory disease complex. Recovered animals may shed the responsible organism for several weeks so any treatment usually continues for three weeks postrecovery. The organism is killed by most disinfectants during routine cleaning.

Vaccination is available, boostered annually.

### *Feline viral respiratory disease*

Also known as:

- Cat flu
- Feline upper respiratory disease (FURD)
- Feline viral rhinotracheitis (FVR)

The two main viruses involved are:

- Feline herpesvirus
- Feline calicivirus

Cats are particularly susceptible to infections (both bacterial and viral) of the nose and throat. Due to their location, these infections are called upper respiratory infections or cat flu. While it is essential to vaccinate, as with the 'human flu', vaccines do not protect against some strains of this disease, especially feline calicivirus.

Calicivirus is easily destroyed outside the host by disinfectants. Transmission of the virus is by aerosol or direct contact. As a result of this, any grouping of cats may lead to infection, i.e. shows, boarding, breeding kennels and veterinary surgeries.

Many cats that have survived the disease become carriers, shedding the virus for several years. It is possible to have suspected carrier animals tested by a veterinary surgeon for the presence of the calicivirus.

The incubation period is up to ten days after exposure to high-risk situations (groups of cats) or stress caused by a change to the environment which may lower the cat's resistance to disease.

Clinical signs include:

- Ulcers on the tongue
- Inflammation of the gums
- Unwilling to eat, but producing excess saliva
- High temperature
- Depressed and listless
- Loss of voice

The presence of ulcers may allow bacteria normally present to add to the cat's original symptoms and recovery time.

Feline herpesvirus can survive outside the host for up to eight days. This virus attacks and replicates in the tissues of the respiratory tract and conjunctiva of the eye, causing viral rhinotracheitis. The tissues from nose (*rhino*) to trachea (*tracheitis*) are affected and inflamed, causing breathing difficulties, sneezing and coughing. Recovered animals can act as carriers, shedding the virus particularly when stressed.

Viral rhinotracheitis is the most serious form of upper respiratory disease, often leaving recovered animals with damage to the nasal passages. This causes the affected cat to periodically sneeze, snuffle and have a runny nose, the discharge occasionally being thick with pus.

The incubation period is from two to ten days postexposure.

Clinical signs include:

- High temperature
- Discharge from eyes and nose, later becoming thickened due to bacterial infection
- Depressed and listless
- Loss of appetite

- Sneezing
- Conjunctivitis
- Mouth ulcers
- Pneumonia
- Abortion in pregnant queens

Vaccine is available, boostered annually by intranasal methods. In high-risk situations, six-monthly administration is advisable.

### Feline infectious anaemia

Infectious anaemia is the direct loss of red blood cells caused by a blood para-site called *Haemobartonella felis or Eperythrozoon felis*. Transmission is thought to be by bloodsucking parasites, e.g. the flea. Cats of all ages can be affected. When the disease is linked to feline leukaemia, affecting white blood cell numbers, the recovery is poor.

The single-celled parasite responsible can be demonstrated on a blood smear examination in the laboratory. Discussion with a veterinary surgeon is essential at this time. Products to safely remove fleas from the affected household are required and other cats in the same household may need to be examined and treated.

Incubation is up to 50 days, with recovered or carrier animals often shedding the parasite for months.

Clinical signs include:

- Pale mucous membranes – mouth and gums
- Breathing difficulty
- Listless and loss of appetite
- Third eyelid up as a sign of ill health
- High temperature
- Weight loss

Animals respond well to treatment using specific antibiotics. There is no vaccine against this virus.

### Feline infectious peritonitis

Also called feline infectious vasculitis, infectious peritonitis is caused by a coronavirus which affects mostly young cats under three years of age. It causes the lining membrane of the abdomen (peritoneum) and contents to become inflamed (peritonitis). This disease is not limited in effect to the organs of the abdomen and may also affect the nervous system and eyes.

Contact between cats via urine and faeces carrying the shed virus will act as the transmission method. Carrier animals may carry the virus for years, with

- Route of administration – subcutaneous or intranasal
- Animal's age
- Medication that could interfere with the vaccine, i.e. anti-inflammatory drugs
- Diet
- Infection already present

Immunity may be acquired by passive or active means. Passive immunity results from the transfer of maternal antibodies to the newborn via the colostrum in the milk. The degree of immunity depends on the quantity of the first milk let down and the quality of the mother's own antibodies resulting from her recent vaccinations. Passive immunity lasts only as long as the antibodies remain active in the blood, from three to 12 weeks. After this time the body will eliminate the antibodies.

Active immunity develops either as a result of the animal becoming infected with a micro-organism, developing the disease and recovering or from a vaccination. Both cause the body to react in much the same manner by stimulating the production of antibodies which are specific to particular microbes (*pathogens* or *antigens*).

Vaccines are prepared from live or inactivated (killed) preparations of micro-organisms. They stimulate the immune system of the vaccinated animal to produce antibodies to specific disease-producing materials.

# Chapter 11
# Zoonones

Also known as zoonoses, these diseases are transmissible from animals to people. Most domestic animals can transmit zoonones.

## Dogs

| Dog infection | Disease in humans |
|---|---|
| Leptospirosis | Weil's disease |
| Toxocariasis | Visceral larval migrans |
| Echinococcosis | Hydatid disease |
| Sarcoptic mange | Skin rash and bites |
| Cheyletiella mites | Skin rash and bites |
| Ringworm | Skin lesions and hair loss |
| Salmonellosis | Diarrhoea/vomiting |
| Rabies | Rabies (hydrophobia) |

## Cats

| Human disease | Signs |
|---|---|
| Pasteurellosis | Bites or scratches become infected |
| Cat scratch fever | High temperature, flu-like signs, rash |
| Ringworm (Fig. 11.1) | Raised, circular, inflamed skin lesion |
| Toxoplasmosis | Abortion of foetus |
| Rabies | Fever, itching at original bite area, behaviour changes, paralysis and death |

## Zoonones from other species

| Disease | Microbe | Species |
|---|---|---|
| Brucellosis | Bacteria | Cattle |
| Campylobacter | Bacteria | Hamsters |

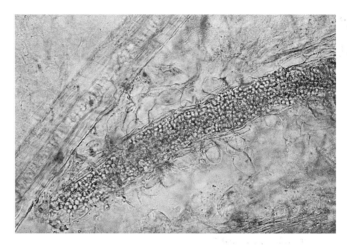

**Fig. 11.1**   Ringworm spores on a hair shaft.

| Psittacosis | Bacteria | Birds |
| Salmonellosis | Bacteria | Mice, rats and guinea pigs |
| Tetanus | Bacteria | Horses and other herbivores |

## Prevention of zoonones

In order to minimise the risk to people of diseases which can be passed by companion animals, the following simple but effective hygiene precautions must be taken:

- Investigate any signs of illness.
- Control fleas and worms.
- Vaccinate animals.
- Do not allow pets to lick children's faces.
- Wash hands after handling any animal.
- Do not feed pets from household plates or dishes.
- Use separate utensils for food preparation.
- Daily collection and safe disposal of faeces.
- Always wear gloves when handling body discharges.

# Chapter 12
# Parasitology

A *parasite* lives in or on another living body. The parasite benefits by taking nourishment from the host, which can be any species.

---

**Parasitology terms**

- *Transport host* – transports the parasite to the next host. No development takes place in the parasite.
- *Paratenic host* – same as transport but the parasite must be eaten, in order to be excreted and passed on to the next host.
- *Intermediate host* – some parasites must spend time on/in this host in order to develop to their next life cycle stage.
- *Final host* – in which the parasite completes its development.
- *Permanent parasite* – develops through all life stages and lives on one host.
- *Temporary parasites* – move from host to host.
- *Endoparasite* – lives inside the host's body.
- *Ectoparasite* – lives on the surface of the host's body.

---

The parasite feeds on the host but does not deliberately kill it as this would destroy its food source. Some hosts may die as a result of the parasite's feeding activities or from toxins released by it

In order to prevent disease or death of the host species, control of parasites is important. Routine control in equine and large animals is necessary to keep parasite numbers down. Control in small animals (dogs, cats, rabbits, etc.) aims to completely remove all parasites, whether internal or external. There are many easy-to-use and effective products for removing external parasites like fleas and lice, with a residue effect which will last for varying periods of time. The products supplied for eliminating internal parasites are collectively called *anthelmintics*.

## External parasites

### Flea – ctenocephalides (Fig. 12.1)

- Adult fleas can live for two years without feeding.
- Flea eggs hatch in 1–2 days.

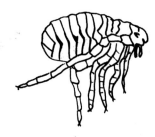

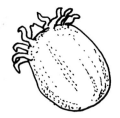

**Fig. 12.2**   Tick – Ixodes.

**Fig. 12.1**   Flea – Ctenocephalides.

- Flea larvae feed for 4–8 days (in carpets or bedding).
- Larvae spin cocoons and adults emerge in five days or less.
- Adult flea cycle may take only three weeks but if the environment is unsuitable, the larval stage can last for months.

## Tick – ixodes (Fig. 12.2)

- Adult tick can live for two years without feeding.
- Engorged female can lay 1000–3000 eggs.
- Larva hatches in 30 days.
- Nymphs emerge from moulted larva.
- Adult tick emerges after 12 days.
- Feeding is required between each stage of development.

## Mite – sarcoptes

Causes sarcoptic mange.

- Sarcoptic mite may live only 3–4 weeks.
- Eggs are laid by the burrowing female (burrows into the epidermal skin layer).
- Larvae hatch in 3–5 days.
- Nymph follows, through two nymph stages.
- Adult mite emerges. The full cycle takes about 17 days.

## Lice

|  | **Dog** | **Cat** |
|---|---|---|
| **Biting louse** | Trichodectes | Felicola substratus |
| **Sucking louse** | Linognathus | |

- Eggs are laid and cemented to the coat hair of the host. Eggs are called *nits*.
- Three stages of nymph emerge.
- Adult emerges after last nymph moult, after three weeks.

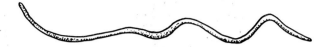

**Fig. 12.3**   Roundworm.

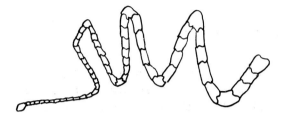

**Fig. 12.4**   Tapeworm.

### *Fur mite – cheyletiella*

- Often referred to as 'walking dandruff'. There are many different types, living on the skin cells and tissue fluid of the host to gain nutrients.
- Eggs are laid and cemented to coat hair, similar to lice.
- Eggs hatch into six-legged larvae.
- Moult into eight-legged larvae.
- Adult stage is reached.

## Internal parasites

Endoparasites for small animals are divided into two groups:

(1)  Roundworms (nematodes) (Fig. 12.3):
  (a)  are unsegmented
  (b)  have body cavity
  (c)  have an alimentary tract throughout.
(2)  Tapeworms (cestodes) (Fig. 12.4):
  (a)  are segmented
  (b)  each segment is independent
  (c)  have a complete alimentary tract in each segment.

  Infected animals do not always show signs of infestation, which only start to appear if the infestation becomes overwhelming to the health of the host animal.

- Scooting on bottom (anal irritation)
- Constantly hungry and eating (*polyphagia*)

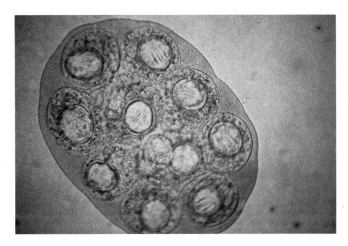

**Fig. 12.5** *Dipylidium caninum* worm egg.

- Weight loss
- Vomiting and diarrhoea seen in heavy infestation
- Unhealthy, dull coat
- Enlarged abdomen

Common worms in the UK include:

- Roundworms
  (a) *Toxocara canis*
  (b) *Toxocara cati*
- Tapeworms
  (a) *Dipylidium caninum*
  (b) *Echinococcus granulosus*

## Life cycles

*Tapeworm – Dipylidium caninum*

This tapeworm affects both dog and cat and has an intermediate host, which is the flea.

(1) Animal passes egg-filled tapeworm segments in its faeces (Fig. 12.5).
(2) The segments burst, releasing individual eggs that are eaten by the flea larvae.
(3) During grooming animal swallows the tapeworm carrying flea larvae.
(4) Tapeworm matures in the animal host.
(5) Adult tapeworm releases mature, egg-filled segments and if not treated with anthelmintic drugs, the cycle begins again.

### Roundworm – Toxocara canis

This worm is a zoonone. It can migrate in human tissues and is linked to blindness in children, a disease called toxocariasis in humans.

(1) Infective eggs or larval forms of this roundworm are swallowed by the dog.
(2) They migrate to the body tissues, often migrating to developing foetuses.
(3) They localise in the intestines, moving to the unborn before the end of pregnancy or infecting them through the mother's milk after birth.
(4) The larvae now mature, passing eggs in the puppies' faeces.
(5) These are swallowed by other puppies or the mother and the cycle repeats unless the dogs are treated.

### Prevention of toxocariasis

- Worm animals regularly.
- Control the intermediate hosts (fleas and lice).
- Dispose of faeces immediately.
- Disinfect where faeces have been.
- Always wash hands thoroughly.
- Wash animal bowls separately from human utensils.
- Do not let animal lick face.
- Keep animal's anal area clean.
- Examine faeces regularly for signs of worms.

# Chapter 13
# Hygiene

## Disinfectants and antiseptics

These chemicals play an important role in maintaining the health and/or promoting the recovery of an animal. Their use in basic hygiene for housing, kennels, catteries or in veterinary practice hospitals is important to the care of both the environment and living tissues. These products are chemicals which, if used incorrectly, such as at low concentrations, allow micro-organisms to develop a resistance, thus reducing their value.

Some of these chemicals are designed for use on the environment and non-living structures, others are designed for use on living tissue.

---

**Hygiene terms**

- *Sterilisation* – the removal or destruction of all living micro-organisms including bacterial spores.
- *Asepsis* – is a state of being free from micro-organisms.
- *Disinfectants* – are referred to as *bactericidal*, i.e. they will kill micro-organisms.
- *Antiseptics* – are referred to as *bacteriostatic*, i.e. they will prevent organisms from multiplying and therefore infections cannot develop.

---

## Principles of disinfection

Disinfectants are used on the environment only, on surfaces like floors, housing walls and ceilings and runs. Disinfectants are harmful to living tissues so if they are used in the workplace or at home, protective clothing (gloves and in some cases masks) should be worn.

Antiseptics are used to disinfect hands prior to operating, before handling animals to prevent transfer of microbes and after handling contaminated material. They are also used to disinfect the patient's skin before and after surgery or after injury.

## *Disinfectants*

Properties of an ideal disinfectant:

- Effective against a wide range of micro-organisms
- Non-toxic to animals or humans
- Non-staining to animals' coats or housing
- Has a good wetting ability and penetrates organic material attached to surfaces
- Stable in storage and has a good shelf-life
- Only low concentrations are necessary for effect
- Economical and readily available

Disinfectants are most effective when:

- Used with hot water rather than cold
- Left in contact with surfaces for the correct amount of time (see instructions on label)
- Used at correct strength
- Not mixed with other chemicals
- Freshly prepared (see instructions on label)

Disinfectants can be inactivated by:

- Organic materials from the body, e.g. blood, faeces, pus and urine
- Surfaces, e.g. cork, wood and plastic
- Materials, e.g. wool or cotton
- Excess minerals in water (hard water areas)
- Mixing disinfectants and detergent

When choosing a disinfectant for the cleaning of housing and surfaces, care is needed. Some products are toxic to certain species of animals. The phenols or phenol-containing compounds are toxic to cats, rabbits and rodents so they tend to be used only in large animal and farming industry facilities. Products in this group are recognised as black, white or clear. They normally have a strong and distinctive smell and will stain housing and bedding materials. Examples are Jeyes Fluid, Izal, Stericol, Ibcol, Phisohex and Dettol.

Disinfectants for environmental use only destroy the micro-organism by disrupting its cell wall or contents in such a way that the microbe will die or be killed by the chemical. The most resistant microbes are:

- Bacterial spores
- Some viruses (unenveloped)

The least resistant microbes are:

- Some viruses (enveloped)
- Bacteria (vegetative)
- Fungi

The most effective disinfectants include:

- Aldehydes
- Peroxides
- Halogens (iodines and chlorines)

### Aldehydes (formaldehyde and glutaraldehyde) (e.g. Formula H, Parvocide and Vetcide)

These are effective against a wide range of micro-organisms but hazardous to living tissue. Never use on living tissues in any form.

Care must be taken while mixing, using and discarding solutions. Avoid contact with skin or eyes and inhaling the fumes. Use these compounds only if necessary and follow work-based safety guidelines for safe use.

### Powdered peroxygen or oxidising agents (peroxides) (e.g. Vircon)

These are effective against a wide range of micro-organisms. They are available in a powder form, which is mixed with water as directed by the manufacturer. The solution is used for disinfection of surfaces and housing. It is considered safe in contact with skin but protective clothes and gloves should be worn, as with all other chemicals. Once mixed, it is stable as a disinfectant for five days. Discard old solution and make up fresh as instructed.

### Halogen group (chlorine release compounds) (e.g. hyperchlorites like household bleach and products like Halamid)

An effective disinfectant if correctly used. Always follow dilution instructions for best effect as this chemical can be inactivated by incorrect dilution and by organic materials.

It is very irritant to tissues so extreme care should be taken in preparation, use and disposal. Thoroughly rinse off any surface that has been in contact with this disinfectant. The product loses activity on exposure to air and light. New dilutions should be made up frequently.

*Iodophors – see antiseptics (Pevidine)*

*Iodine*

This is used on surfaces as a solution of water or alcohol. It is effective against a wide range of micro-organisms but can be inactivated by organic matter. It will also stain surfaces and materials.

## Antiseptics (used as skin cleaners)

When applied to skin or mucous membranes of living tissues, antiseptics stop or prevent the growth of micro-organisms like bacteria and fungi but will not necessarily kill microbes.

*Quaternary ammonium compounds (QACs) (a) chlorhexidine plus a detergent property, e.g. Hibiscrub or Dinex; (b) cetrimide, e.g. Cetavlon, Savlon or Vetasep*

These are effective against microbes and have a rapid action as an antiseptic. They are often used as a preoperative skin cleaner and as a surgeon's scrub. They have a low toxicity to tissues but may be irritant to some individuals. Recontamination by microbes is prevented for a time due to a residual effect. Use at recommended dilution and only on intact skin.

*Iodophors – iodine-based compounds (e.g. Pevidine scrub, Betadine)*

These are effective against skin microbes, non-irritant and have low toxicity to tissues. Their action is slow so length of time in contact with the skin surface is important. Follow instructions for use.

# Disinfecting housing or surfaces

To maximise the effect of the chemicals being used and to prevent inactivation by organic materials, the following rules apply:

(1)   Remove animal, food bowls, toys and bedding.
(2)   Soak all surfaces with hot, soapy water.
(3)   Scrub the soaked surfaces with bristle brush.
(4)   Wash and rinse away all materials and soap.
(5)   Apply the disinfectant at correct dilution and for correct time.
(6)   Rinse all trace of disinfectant off with water and hose down.
(7)   Leave to dry.

# Chapter 14
# Basic Nutrition

Food or nutrients are required by the body in order to produce energy. Energy is necessary to drive the essential processes and systems in the body.

- Breathing
- Circulating the blood to tissues and cells
- Maintaining body temperature
- Muscle movement throughout the body
- The materials for repair, growth and reproduction
- General health

Nutrients are any food product which will support life. There are six major groups:

- Those which supply energy:
  - (1) protein
  - (2) carbohydrates
  - (3) fats
- Those which do not supply energy but are needed for its production:
  - (4) vitamins
  - (5) minerals
  - (6) water

Animals eat in order to satisfy their energy needs. In the wild, when animals have eaten enough food to meet the body's energy demands, they will stop. However, due to the improved taste of pet foods, scraps from the human table and 'treats', some companion animals will eat in excess of their body's needs resulting in obesity and other linked diseases. Many animals have a sedentary lifestyle with owners unable to provide sufficient exercise which means that nutrients in excess of body needs will be converted to storage as body fat (*adipose tissue*).

# Protein

(a)   Animal origin
- Meat
- Fish
- Eggs
- Milk

(b)   Vegetable origin
- Soya and other pulses/beans
- Cereals

Proteins are large molecules, consisting of hundreds of single units called *amino acids* which join together as chains. Dietary protein is broken down during the digestive process into amino acids. Proteins are made up of a combination of 23 amino acids. Animals need all 23 amino acids in order to maintain their body proteins. Some are obtained from food and some are made within the body.

Dogs require ten amino acids to be supplied by the diet and can create or synthesise the remainder. Cats require 11 amino acids to be supplied via the diet. The extra one cannot be synthesised by the cat and can only be obtained from animal protein. These dietary amino acids are referred to as *essential*.

## Function

- Energy (only used as energy if in excess or other energy sources not available)
- Growth
- Repair of tissues
- Immune system to protect from disease
- Assisting metabolic reactions (enzyme and hormone)

## Deficiency

- Poor growth
- Weight loss
- Disease

Many tissues in the body rely on protein as a major component, e.g. hormones, enzymes, plasma proteins and antibodies. The quantities required by each animal will vary depending on:

- Species
- Age

- Sex
- Quality of the protein

The higher the biological value of a protein (in other words, the easier it is for the body to use), the smaller the quantity required. High-value protein includes:

- Egg
- White meat (chicken)
- Fish

Low-value protein includes:

- Soya bean and other pulses
- Cereals

Excess protein in the diet cannot be stored but is converted by the liver to energy and nitrogenous waste (urea). This is then removed from the body by the kidneys.

## Carbohydrate

(a) Animal origin
  - Milk
(b) Vegetable origin
  - Cereal starches (oats, lentils, rice)
  - Root vegetables (potatoes)

Carbohydrate can be divided into digestible (starches) and indigestible (dietary fibre or cellulose). It is found in plants and cereals and provides bulk to the faecal materials. It assists in regulating bowel function and the movement of undigested nutrients through the digestive tract.

### Function

- Energy
- Provides dietary fibre

### Deficiency

- None, providing other energy nutrients are available in the diet (i.e. fats or proteins)

Carbohydrate is broken down in the digestive tract to simple sugars which are essential for most of the body's energy. If simple sugars are unavailable as a nutrient the body can divert some amino acids to become an energy source.

If the diet contains more carbohydrate than required in the production of energy, the surplus is converted into body fat and stored as adipose tissue.

Simple sugars can be converted into a temporary stored form called *glycogen*. This is stored in the liver and muscles and converted back to simple sugar whenever its energy is needed by the body.

# Fats

(a)  Animal origin
  •  Milk and other dairy produce
  •  Fish oil
  •  Fat of body origin (attached to meat)
(b)  Vegetable origin
  •  Nuts
  •  Seed oils, i.e. sunflower, oil seed rape, linseed
  •  Margarine

## *Function*

•  Energy (a very concentrated form)
•  Improved taste to the diet
•  For the absorption, transport and storage of the fat-soluble vitamins – A, D, E and K
•  Provide essential fatty acids for body use

## *Deficiency*

•  Reproduction problems
•  Impaired wound healing
•  Poor coat condition
•  Dry skin

Fat is also called *lipid*. It is made up of glycerol, with attached fatty acids. Fatty acids are a very concentrated form of energy compared to protein or carbohydrates.

In the dog and cat there are three essential fatty acids: linoleic, arachidonic and linolenic. Provided there is a dietary source, the dog can obtain or synthesise all three from any type of dietary fat. The cat, however, is only able to synthesise one essential fatty acid from the diet and must therefore be provided with a

**Table 14.1** Fat-soluble vitamins.

| Vitamin | Source | Function |
|---|---|---|
| A (retinol) | Fish oils, liver, egg and cereals | Night vision, body cell division |
| D (cholecalciferol) | Liver, fish oils, egg and cereals | Regulates calcium levels, bone growth and repair |
| E (tocopherol) | Vegetable oils, egg and cereals | Supports tissues and cells around the body |
| K | Developed in the intestines (no need for dietary source), green vegetables | Assists in blood clotting |

**Table 14.2** Water-soluble vitamins.

| Vitamin | Source | Function |
|---|---|---|
| $B_1$ (thiamine) | Cereals, organ meat, green vegetables, dairy products | Assists metabolic, reactions, i.e. converts sugars to fatty tissues |
| $B_2$ (riboflavin) | Organ meats, milk | Use and release of energy by cells |
| $B_6$ (pyridoxine) | Cereals, meat and yeast | Metabolism of amino acids |
| $B_{12}$ (cyanocobalamin) | Fish, organ meats | Blood cell production in bone marrow |
| Folic acid | Organ meats, fish. Synthesised by gut | Blood cell production in bone marrow |
| Biotin | Produced by gut bacteria | Assists body metabolism |
| C | Green vegetables | Creates collagen for tissues |
| Ascorbic acid | Created in the body | Supports bone cells |

Dogs and cats may synthesise most vitamin C required by the body but primates, fish and guinea pigs are unable to do so and must receive a dietary source for body health and function.

dietary source of the other two. Combined with the need to be supplied with one of the amino acids in the dietary food, this means the cat is considered a true carnivore. That is, it cannot maintain full health without a dietary source of animal tissues to utilise as a ready-made essential fat or amino acid.

Body fat (adipose tissue) is created from a combination of fatty acids and simple sugars, if either is in excess in the diet.

# Vitamins

Vitamins are important in the chemical reactions that go to make up metabolism. There are two groups:

- Fat-soluble vitamins – A, D, E and K (Table 14.1)
- Water-soluble vitamins – B complex group and vitamin C (Table 14.2)

Fat-soluble vitamins are stored in fatty tissues and in the liver; and therefore could reach dangerous levels if given in excess. Water-soluble vitamins are not stored and must be continuously supplied via the diet and supplemented in medical conditions that lead to water loss, i.e. diarrhoea. Most species can produce vitamin C in the liver but the guinea pig cannot and must be supplemented as a routine.

## Minerals

(a)  Animal origin
  • Dairy products
  • Meat
  • Egg
  • Bone meal
(b)  Vegetable origin
  • Cereals
  • Green vegetables
  • Salt

These are important for a variety of functions in the body. They are often referred to as *ash* on containers of pet food.

Providing the animal is fed a balanced dietary product, minerals do not normally need to be supplemented.

Minerals are divided into two groups:

(1)  Macro or major minerals (needed in large or regular amounts):
  • calcium
  • chloride
  • magnesium
  • phosphorus
  • potassium
  • sodium
(2)  Trace minerals (needed in only small amounts):
  • copper
  • iodine
  • iron
  • selenium
  • zinc

### *Function*

  • Assist maintenance of pH balance in the body
  • Maintain the body's fluid balance

- Essential for the function of muscle tissues and conducting nerve impulses
- Help regulate the body's metabolism (via enzymes and hormones)

Never feed any one product in excess within an otherwise balanced diet. Deficiencies in minerals are often associated with excess minerals being added to the diet, i.e. calcium deficiencies can be caused by phosphorus excess in the diet. This could happen in animals being fed an excess of dietary meat or organ tissues.

## Water

Sixty to 70% of body weight is water. Water is essential for all cells in the body and is found inside and outside all cells. It is involved with nearly every body process. As a result of the presence of water in the body, the following can take place:

- Transport of any material between tissues/cells
- Electrolyte balance
- pH balance
- Control of temperature
- Lubrication of all tissue cells
- A medium for blood and lymph

Unfortunately water cannot be stored by the body and must be available all the time for all animals. Water in the body comes from:

- Food
- Drinking
- Chemical reactions (metabolism)

Water is lost:

- In urine
- Via the lungs in breathing
- In faeces
- In sweat via the skin

It is important to stress that *fresh water must be available at all times*. This must be emphasised to all pet owners. Some water will be available from canned food but if a dry diet is given, the animal must receive water by drinking.

## General considerations for feeding

- There are major differences in the dietary needs of each species of animal.
- If the diet is balanced for that species, do not supplement vitamins or minerals.
- The diet should provide enough energy for the animal, supplied by fats and carbohydrate rather than by diverting protein.
- Energy levels and requirements will vary with age or life stages and activity levels.
- Read instructions carefully before feeding dry diets in particular. Use a recommended 'measure' for quantities to prevent overfeeding.

# Chapter 15
# Handling

It is necessary to appreciate the behavioural differences between species in order to perform handling safely. Body language is quite complex in some species, i.e. the dog, and must be taken into account before approaching.

Handling may give rise to fear and stress in the animal, which may be a learned response after a bad handling experience. Any knowledge of the individual's temperament or behaviour in given situations and previous required handling is helpful information.

## Reasons for handling

- Daily and weekly checks
- Grooming
- Transportation
- First aid situation
- Examination after injury
- Medicating

Animals should be accustomed to handling from an early age. Teaching the animal to tolerate having difficult areas, such as ears, feet and mouth, looked at will make life less stressful for animal and handler at a later date.

## Approaching to handle

- Assess animal's behaviour and body language.
- Be quiet but confident to establish dominance of the situation.
- Talk in a reassuring manner.
- Never corner the animal; always leave supposed choices.
- With a dog or cat, reach out to introduce yourself to the animal.
- Stroke the animal and accustom it to voice and scent.
- Only lift the animal if the approach has been accepted.
- Handle with minimum restraint, especially cats.
- If the animal becomes or is aggressive, then a firm method of restraint is needed for the safety of handlers.

---

**Behaviour seen when animals are unwilling to be handled**

- *Cats* – hiss, adopt defensive posture, growl, strike with front claws and flatten their ears to the skull.
- *Dogs* – hackles raised, growling, lips in snarl position, ears forward, barking and attempting to bite.
- *Rabbits* – biting, scratching using hind legs, thumping hind legs on floor and, if terrified, squealing.
- *Guinea pigs* – are not aggressive but will stampede or circle their housing in an effort to get away.
- *Rats* – bite if startled or hurt.

---

## Holding procedures

### Rat

Place hand firmly over back and rib cage, restrain head with thumb and forefinger immediately behind lower jaw (Figs 15.1 and 15.2).

### Guinea pig

Grasp under the trunk with one hand while supporting the hindquarters with the other hand (Fig. 15.3).

### Gerbil

Never lift by the middle or end of the tail. The tail is firmly grasped at the base and the gerbil is lifted and cradled in the palm of the hand. Use the over-the-back grip to prevent struggling (Figs 15.4 and 15.5).

### Rabbit

Never lift using only the ears.

- *Short distances* (for cleaning housing) – grasp the skin over the neck with one hand and support the hindquarters with the other (Fig. 15.6).
- *Longer distances* – having lifted the rabbit from housing using the above method, it is positioned against the handler with its head tucked under the handler's arm, the hindquarters being supported by the handler's arms (Fig. 15.7).

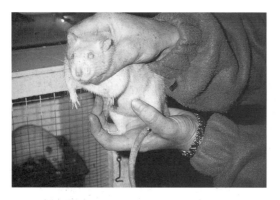

**Fig. 15.1** Correct holding technique for a rat.

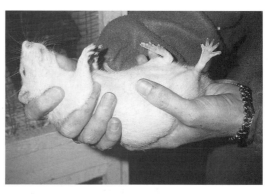

**Fig. 15.2** Correct holding technique to expose the abdomen and chest.

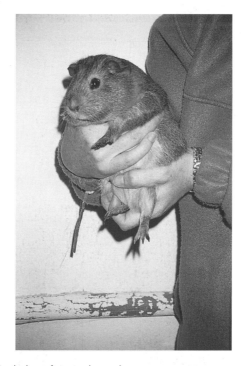

**Fig. 15.3** Holding technique for a guinea pig.

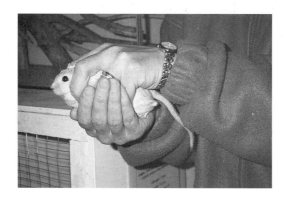

**Fig. 15.4** Holding a gerbil.

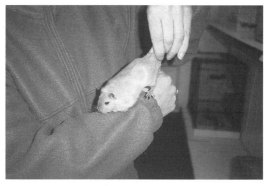

**Fig. 15.5** Restraint for a gerbil.

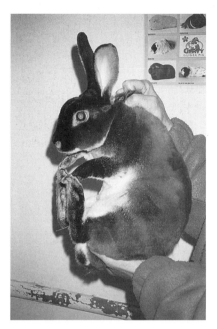

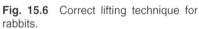

**Fig. 15.6**  Correct lifting technique for rabbits.

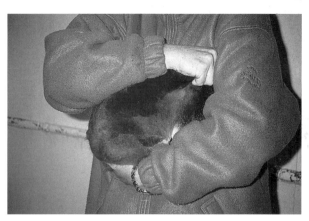

**Fig. 15.7**  Correct technique for moving a rabbit longer distances.

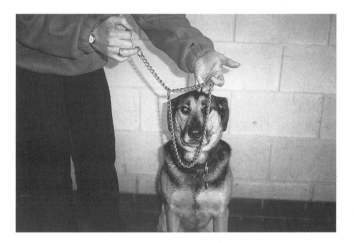

**Fig. 15.8**  Check chain position – correct size and correctly held.

## *Dog*

Before handling, always check the following:

- The collar is correctly fitted and will not slip off.
- Position of check chain (correct size/correct fit) (Fig. 15.8).
- Temperament (muzzle if necessary).
- Reason for handling.

**To tape muzzle a dog**

Two handlers are required, one to hold the dog and one to apply the muzzle.

*Dog handler*

- Stands facing the same way as the dog and to one side (alongside the shoulder).
- Takes hold of the scruff and collar (if worn) with both hands, behind the dog's ears.

*Person applying tape muzzle*

- Use a bandage which will not stretch.
- Cut a length in excess to requirements.
- Make a loop with a double throw knot (Fig. 15.9).

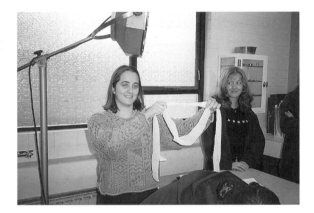

**Fig. 15.9**   Make a loop with the tape muzzle, with a double throw knot.

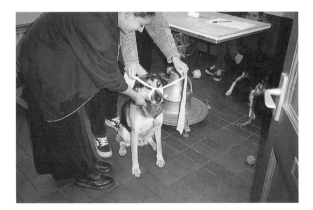

**Fig. 15.10**   Drop the loop over the dog's mouth and nose and tighten the loop.

*Continued*

**To tape muzzle a dog** (*Continued*)

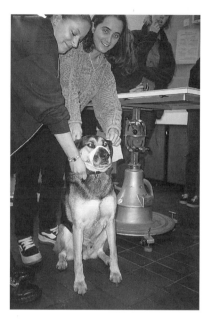

**Fig. 15.11**    Knot the ends behind the ears and tie a bow for quick release.

- Keeping the loop open, approach from the side of the dog.
- Drop the loop over the dog's mouth and nose and tighten the loop quickly (Fig. 15.10).
- Cross the muzzle ties under the jaw.
- Knot the ends behind the dog's ears and tie into a bow for quick release (Fig. 15.11).

# Restraint procedures in the dog and cat

## *For intravenous injection*

Presenting one of the forelegs for procedures such as an injection into the vein or taking a blood sample (Figs 15.12, 15.13 and 15.14).

### On its side (lateral position)

To expose the limbs, chest or abdomen (Fig. 15.18).

### For general examinations

In these situations, the head must be controlled (Figs 15.19 and 15.20).

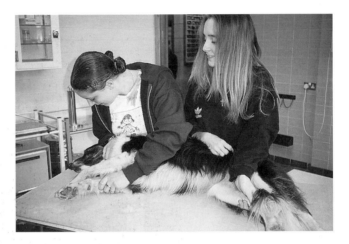

**Fig. 15.18**    Restraint for access to limbs, chest or abdomen.

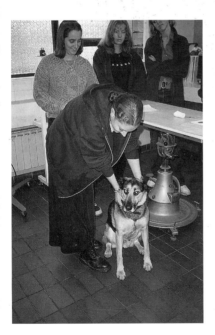

**Fig. 15.19**    Controlling the head standing to the side.

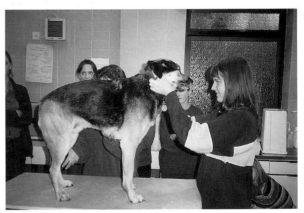

**Fig. 15.20**    Controlling the head standing in front.

**Approaching a cat**

- Use calm, confident movements.
- Speak quietly all the time.
- Attempt to stroke the head first and then along the cat's back.
- When the cat responds (non-aggressively)
- Pick the cat up (Fig. 15.21).

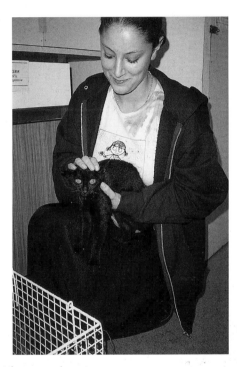

**Fig. 15.21**   Lifting cat from carrying cage.

**Transferring a cat from basket to examination table or surface**

- Place one hand under the chest and, supporting the hindquarters, lift.
- Hold under one arm, hand still under the chest, and transfer other hand to support and control the cat's head.
- Alternatively, this hand could scruff the neck to control the head.
- Never overrestrain a cat unless really necessary.

# Chapter 16
# Grooming and Coat Care

One of the many responsibilities of a dog or cat owner is that of coat care. As breeds of dog and cat were developed for size, character and colour, so their coat length, texture and density evolved. Careful management of these many and varied coat types is part of the owner/pet interaction. Often, the choice of breed is based on a dog or cat seen in a breed book but it is essential to investigate the amount of time and frequency of coat care required. There is a vast difference in the time it takes to groom a Doberman and an Old English Sheepdog, a Siamese and a Persian cat.

---

**Main aims of grooming**

- Remove dead hair
- Clean the skin
- Clean the coat
- Remove knots and tangles

---

## Dogs

Grooming covers the following factors:

- Bonding
- Trust
- Accustoms the pet to handling
- Information on the condition of the skin
- Presence of external parasites (fleas or mites)
- Monitoring of nail condition
- General health status information

### The coat

The earliest breeds of dog evolved in the northern hemisphere and so needed a dense coat for protection from the cold. As dogs moved further south to the warmer climates of the world, their coat became thinner and shorter to allow the

Examples of coat type in the dog.

| Type | Hair length | Breeds | Grooming frequency |
|------|-------------|--------|--------------------|
| Smooth (Fig. 16.1) | Short and fine | Chihuahua | Minimal grooming |
| | | Boxer | Twice weekly |
| | | Doberman | Weekly |
| | | Whippet | Weekly |
| | | Pointer | Weekly |
| | Long and dense | Labrador | Twice weekly |
| | | Corgi | Weekly |
| Double (Fig. 16.2) | Medium to long | Collie | Daily and weekly |
| | | German Shepherd | Daily and weekly |
| | | Old English Sheepdog | Daily and weekly |
| Wiry (Fig. 16.3) | Short | Dachshund | Weekly |
| | | West Highland White | Weekly |
| | Long | Airedale | Daily and weekly |
| | | Schnauzer | Daily and weekly |
| Silky (Fig. 16.4) | Short | Spaniel | Daily and weekly |
| | | Pekinese | Daily and weekly |
| | Long | Afghan | Daily and weekly |
| | | Yorkshire | Daily and weekly |
| Woolly/curly (Fig. 16.5) | | Bedlington | Daily and weekly |
| | | Poodle | Daily and weekly |
| | | Kerry Blue | Daily and weekly |

*Daily* indicates the coat should be briefly groomed once a day.
*Weekly* means the coat should be thoroughly groomed once a week.

dog to function in extreme heat. Selective breeding further enhanced coat features for specific breeds and purposes. The table above shows different coat types.

Every breed varies in the type of coat hair it has. Hairs grow in hair follicles with several hairs to each follicle. Usually there is an outer coat composed of *primary* or *guard hairs* and an undercoat made up of secondary hairs. Often the undercoat is finer than the outer coat.

Hair will be shed periodically. The growth rate of hair varies from breed to breed. Other factors which influence the growth of hair are as follows.

### Seasons

- *Spring* – triggers production of the summer coat, causing the old winter coat to be shed. The coat is oily, due to an increase in the sebaceous gland activity in the skin.
- *Autumn* – triggers the production of the much denser winter coat, causing the summer coat to be shed. The coat is less oily due to reduced sebaceous gland activity.

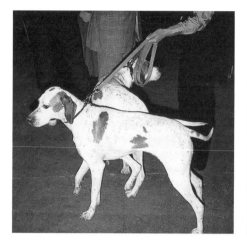

**Fig. 16.1** Smooth coat – Pointer.

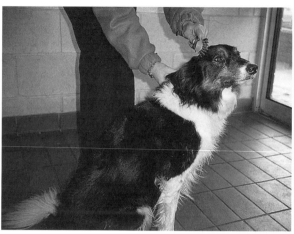

**Fig. 16.2** Double coat – Collie.

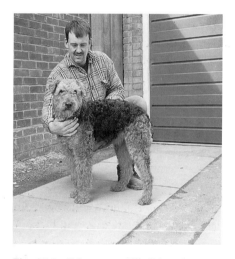

**Fig. 16.3** Wire coat – Airedale.

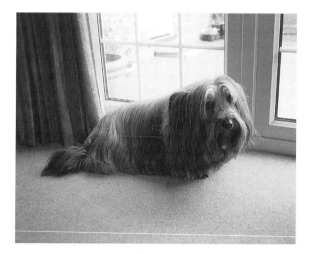

**Fig. 16.4** Silky coat – Skye Terrier.

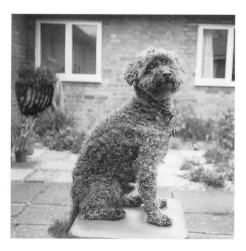

**Fig. 16.5** Woolly/curly coat – Poodle.

*Environmental temperature*

Dogs kept in centrally heated housing will shed their coat continuously. Dogs kept in outside kennels will shed in spring and autumn.

*Ill health*

If the animal becomes debilitated due to acute or chronic illness the coat growth cycle will be interrupted.

*Diet*

A balanced diet with all essential nutrients will ensure normal coat growth and condition.

*Hormone levels*

Levels will alter during oestrus in the bitch, slowing the rate of growth. The coat texture can alter in some disease conditions which affect the body's hormone levels, not only causing the coat to grow more slowly but also making it coarse and rough to touch.

## Grooming notes

*Smooth coat*

Matting of this type of coat does not occur due to its short length. However, the coat will become clogged with dead hair when moulting. Increased grooming at this time will keep the skin in good condition. To prevent loss of natural oils in the coat, only bath if really necessary. If the coat is muddy, brush it out once the coat is dry.

Equipment required:

- *Short coat* – use a hound glove
- *Long coat* – use a comb and a bristle brush

*Double coat*

Will matt and tangle if not groomed frequently. Regular grooming sessions of up to three-quarters of an hour to one hour may be necessary to prevent the coat tangling. Some breeds in this category, for example the Old English Sheepdog, are clipped to about 2.5 cm in length in order to simplify grooming. This summer clip will allow the dog to cope better in hot weather.

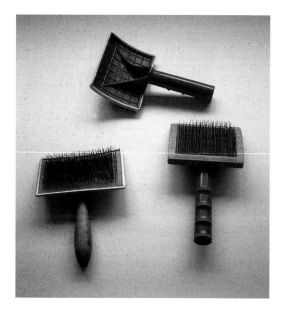

**Fig. 16.6** Slicker/carder brushes.

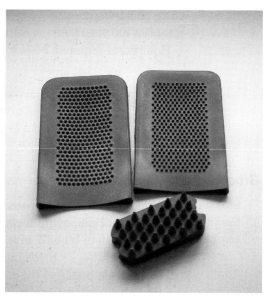

**Fig. 16.7** Hound glove (top) and rubber brush (below).

ing the skin surface, are set in a flexible rubber-backed cushion. The pin brush will separate hairs and lay the coat in position, particularly useful for the silky long coats and double coats. These brushes also stimulate the skin, distributing the natural oils from the skin to the tips of the hairs. If the coat has tangled hair or knots, then use a comb first to remove these before brushing. This will prevent the coat being pulled or broken when the pin brush is used.

*Slicker/carder brushes* (Fig. 16.6), with a wooden or rigid plastic handle, come in a range of sizes. The pins are hooked and set in a rubber-backed cushion, giving some flexibility to the grooming movement. The function of these hooked pins is to remove dead coat. No pressure should be applied when using the slicker brush because the pins could easily scratch or damage the skin surface. It can be used on a range of coat types from silky to double and in some body areas of curly and wire-coated breeds. Never use on areas of the body where the coat is normally thin such as the stomach, groin or armpits.

A *hound glove* (Fig. 16.7) fits over the groomer's hand like a mitten or glove, as the name suggests. It is made of flexible plastic or rubber with short bristles made from wire or plastic and some have a velvet-type surface on one side and bristles on the other. It is used to remove dead or moulting hair (bristle side) and to polish the coat (velvet side) in smooth and short-coated breeds. Care should be taken when using the bristle side, in case too much pressure is used and the skin is damaged.

### Combs

Combs are used to remove dead hair and prevent mats forming behind the ears, in the neck/collar area and over the hindquarters.

Combs are available in metal or plastic, with or without handles (Fig. 16.8). Some combs are half wide toothed and half fine toothed so that each half can be used in different body areas and on different coat types. The teeth tips are rounded or plastic coated to avoid tearing the skin surface. Some combs also have pins set so that they are able to roll individually and prevent coat damage when in contact with a mat or tangle.

Combs should be used carefully, especially when encountering a knot or tangle. Slowly tease the hairs and never rush this stage or the coat will be pulled, hurting the dog and making it unwilling to be groomed.

*Rake combs* (Fig. 16.9) have ridged metal teeth with round tips, set perpendicular to the handle, and resemble a small garden rake. They should not be used by pressing into the coat. Their function is to break up mats and, in dense coats, lift and remove dead undercoat hair. They are pulled towards the groomer through the coat and in the direction of the coat hair.

*Flea combs* have fine teeth set close together, with a grip area. These are pulled slowly and carefully through the coat, going with the normal coat direction. If a parasite is encountered, the gap between the teeth is too small for it to pass through so it is lifted onto the comb for the groomer to remove.

*Dematting combs* (Fig. 16.10) have wooden handles and teeth which on one side are rounded and blunt and on the other side are a series of cutting blades. These combs are used, with extreme care, to cut through large mats of hair by placing the blunt side against the dog's skin surface and with a gentle sawing action cutting away from the skin surface and through the mat. This will allow the matted areas to either be combed out or further subdivided for combing and removal of the dead hair.

### Cutting equipment

A *stripping knife or comb* (Fig. 16.11) is used to remove dead hair and at the same time trim the live hair. The comb has a serrated metal cutting edge, set against a guard plate on one side for the removal of dead hair. The stripping knife has a metal handle and blade. Sections of coat hair are held between the operator's thumb and the blade and the blade is pulled away from the skin with a twisting movement. At the same time, dead hair can be pulled or plucked. This is known as hand stripping and is used on wire-coated breeds such as terriers, wire-coated Dachshunds and Schnauzers. If done correctly, it is not at all painful.

*Thinning scissors* (Fig. 16.12) have one regular and one serrated blade or both blades serrated. They thin the coat without affecting its appearance. These scissors are therefore used on the undercoat, preserving the colour of the outer coat appearance.

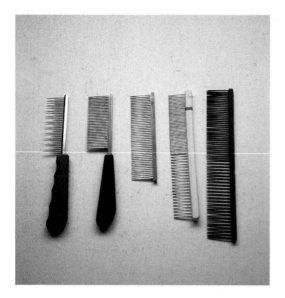

**Fig. 16.8** Comb types.

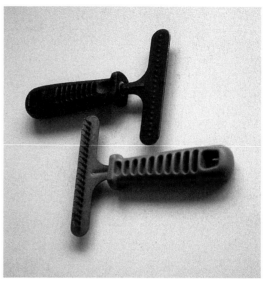

**Fig. 16.9** Rake comb.

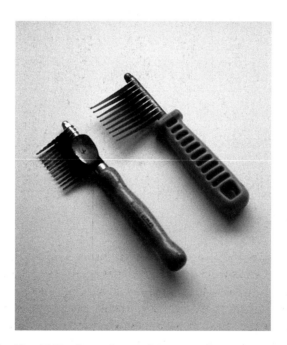

**Fig. 16.10** Dematting comb.

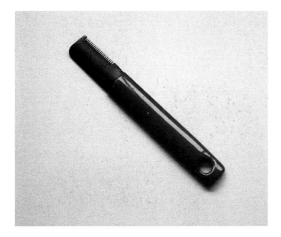

**Fig. 16.11** Stripping knife.

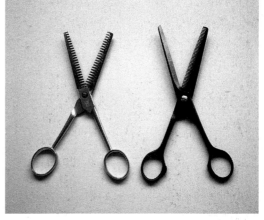

**Fig. 16.12** Thinning scissors or shears.

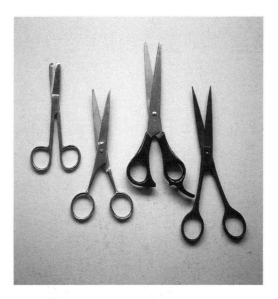

**Fig. 16.13** Scissor types.

*Scissors* (Fig. 16.13) are available in many sizes and shapes for use on the various body areas, from long, sharp, tapering blades to short, blunt-ended blades, depending on the area that requires a trim. Blunt-ended scissors are used to trim between toes and in delicate areas around the eyes, ears, lips and genitals.

*Electric clippers* (Fig. 16.14) are used by professional groomers in conjunction with scissors, particularly in the curly-coated breeds such as the poodle. These coats keep growing all year round and need constant attention. Always keep the blade of the clippers flat to the coat to avoid cutting the skin.

The clipper cuts away the excess hair more rapidly than scissors and is used with a variety of detachable blades. The blades vary from fine tooth for close

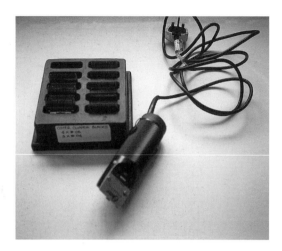

**Fig. 16.14** Electric clipper with range of blades.

trims to ones set with wide-spaced blades or teeth, which leave short hairs against the skin surface. The blades are snapped onto a post on the clipper only when the clipper is running.

The clipper is held like a pencil which gives a firm grip, allowing the groomer to move over the coat lightly and keep the blade flat against the section being clipped.

Clippers will get hot during use so it is important to closely monitor the blade temperature in order to prevent a clipper burn or rash developing on the damaged skin surface. There are several ways of avoiding this:

- Spray hot blades with aerosol lubricant spray to reduce temperature.
- Change the hot blade for a new cool blade.
- Use a second clipper, allowing the first to cool.
- Keep the blades in use sharpened.
- Only clip hair that is completely dry.

*Nail clippers* (Fig. 16.15) are only used to cut nails which are overlong. A range of clippers is available, from the guillotine clipper (also useful in small mammals) to the double blade type. The choice of nail clipper will depend on the length and position of the nail presented.

## Grooming procedure

Depending on the coat type of a dog, grooming will be a daily and/or a weekly event. It provides the owner with the opportunity not only to condition the coat and skin but to:

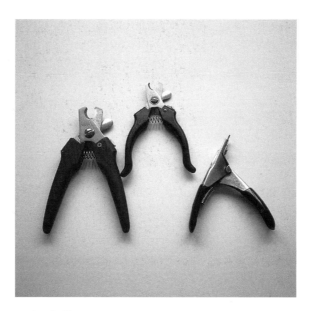

**Fig. 16.15** Types of nail clippers.

- Clean any discharge and examine the eyes
- Check and clean the ear to prevent infection developing
- Clean and examine the mouth and particularly the teeth
- Examine and trim any overlong toe nails
- Check the anal region

*Eyes* should be bright and free of any discharge. If any discharge is seen in the corner of the eye, moisten a clean piece of cotton wool with water and wipe away in the direction of the nose. If the discharge looks anything other than clear, check for signs of inflammation and seek veterinary attention.

*Ears* should be free of wax, a dull pink colour and without odour. In the curly-coated breeds, the ears need to be plucked free of hair which, if left in place, attracts wax, parasites and infection. Check for signs of discomfort or reluctance by the dog when the flap is being examined, which may indicate a problem.

*Mouth.* The gums and tongue should be pink (pigmented in the Chow chow) or partly pink with pigmented areas. Gums should be well defined around each tooth, with no food or other materials attached. In order to prevent any build-up of tartar on the teeth, pet toothpaste in various flavours and tooth brushes can be used as part of the daily grooming examination.

*Feet* or paws should be clean around the nail bed, nails just in contact with the ground, excess hair cut short between the pads and nails to prevent mats and grass seed barbs penetrating the skin and causing an abscess.

*Anal region* under the tail and around the anus needs to be checked daily in dogs, whether short or long coated. The area should be free of any faecal material and show no signs of redness or inflammation. Should the dog start licking excessively around the anal region or scooting on its rear end, the anal glands should be checked for a blockage. These glands are situated on either side of the anus and may not empty as expected when the dog defecates, leading to infection.

### Nail clipping

Active healthy dogs do not need frequent nail clips. The nails will wear naturally with everyday use. The exception may be the dew claw, which can grow round into the nail bed if left unchecked, although they tend to be slow growing in most breeds.

The nails may need attention if:

- The dog is exercised only on soft ground or grass
- The dog is elderly
- Due to limb injury, the dog walks with uneven gait
- A nail becomes broken or damaged

### Technique

(1)  Restrain and reassure dog during the procedure.
(2)  Inspect each foot, identifying which nails need attention.
(3)  Locate the 'quick' (the nerve and blood supply).
(4)  Cut below the quick.
(5)  Smooth any rough edges with a nail file.

In some dogs the nails are pigmented, making it impossible to see the quick. In these cases always be cautious and cut less to avoid damage to the quick. If still unsure of the amount to be clipped, seek instruction from a groomer or a veterinary practice. Once a dog has had a bad experience during nail clipping, it will never forget, making future occasions difficult for the handler.

### Brushing the coat

Once the general checks are complete, brushing and combing in preparation for the bath can begin. It is essential to brush and comb before the bath to remove all matted and tangled hair. Shampoo and drying make matting much worse in some coat types. Comb check the coat to ensure no tangles are left.

Start the procedure with:

(1)  The hind legs
(2)  Then the forelegs
(3)  Back to the tail section and tail

(4)   The body coat, one side at a time

(5)   Chest area

(6)   Lastly the head, face and ears

Pay particular attention to the groin area and the armpit area on the forelegs where mats may develop. The head and ears in breeds such as Poodle, Cocker Spaniel, Lhasa Apso and Afghan need particular attention. The ear hair is long and fine and tends to form small mats.

The eye area on breeds such as Pekinese and Shih Tzu needs particular attention and care and these are short-nosed breeds (*brachycephalic*) with protruding eyes. As a last resort, it may be necessary to remove mats and tangles with scissors or electric clippers, especially if it is clearly painful to the dog or the dog is becoming aggressive due to the grooming.

### Bathing

Reasons for bathing:

- To control skin parasites
- To clean soiled coat
- To remove odours
- To improve coat appearance for showing
- As part of a medical treatment
- To mask the scent of oestrus

Equipment includes:

- Cotton wool to plug ears (optional)
- Shampoo/conditioner
- Mixer hose or jug
- Bath with non-slip mat
- Towel or dryer

*Ear plugs.* After brushing and combing, ear plugs may be placed in the ear canal to prevent the entry of shampoo and water. This is optional and should not be used if upsetting to the dog.

*Shampoo.* Use a general-purpose shampoo unless the coat requires otherwise. Conditioners may be used to improve the coat texture and make it more manageable for final brushing when dry.

Shampoos available include the following:

- *Mild* – have only low levels of detergent to avoid eye or skin irritation.
- *Medicated* – prescribed by a veterinary surgeon in cases where the dog has

skin problems. These shampoos contain antiseptics such as iodine to reduce skin bacteria levels or drugs to assist a specific skin condition.

- *Insecticidal* – for control of surface/skin parasites such as lice, fleas and ticks. These are often used in combination with parasite control programmes that use spot on, tablet or injection methods.
- *Colour enhancing* – used to improve the appearance of coats, particularly white ones.
- *Conditioners* – used to prevent tangles in long-haired coats and improve the brushing-out process once dry. Used in show dogs such as Yorkshire Terriers, Maltese Terriers, Afghans and Shih Tzus.

Always decant the shampoo required into a plastic container (such as an old washing-up liquid bottle) as this allows easy application of the shampoo, used either concentrated or diluted. If the shampoo should be knocked and fall there is no risk of broken glass and the noise of the container falling will not frighten the dog.

*Mixer hose or jug.* Use of a hose with a shower head allows the water pressure and temperature to be regulated (Fig. 16.16). If a hose is not available for rinsing, then use a jug.

*Bath.* A household bath can be used, with a hair catcher over the plug hole to prevent blockage, or a child's paddling pool. Always provide a non-slip surface to prevent the dog from damaging the bath surface if it slips or panics. Rubber bath mats or car mats can be used.

*Towels or dryer.* Several towels are needed for any breed other than small or toy (Fig. 16.17). Always provide more than required to avoid having to leave a half-dry dog to shake off the excess water over all surfaces. In winter, place the dog in a warm area to dry once excess water has been removed from the coat using towels. Household hand-held hair dryers (Fig. 16.18) may be used but be careful introducing the dog to the dryer as the noise and warm air flow may frighten it. Never hold dryers too close or use a high-temperature high-flow setting.

- *Floor dryers* – mounted on stands, are powerful, quickly drying heavy-coated breeds (Figs 16.19 and 16.20).
- *Cage dryers* – attach to the front of holding kennels and cages. These are used after towel drying.
- *Wall-mounted dryers* – similar to the hand-held dryer but more powerful and space saving. A hose applies the 'blow dry' effect when directed on to the dog's coat.
- *Cabinet dryers* (Fig. 16.21) box cages with a false, vented floor, containing the blow dryer. Warm air flows, fan assisted, into the box area where the dog sits.

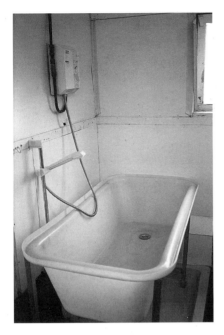

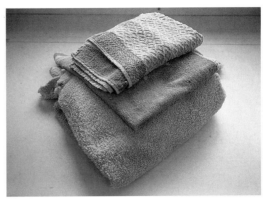

**Fig. 16.17**   Have several towels available.

**Fig. 16.16**   Dog bath with shower hose.

*Method of bathing.* Make sure before bathing starts that all the equipment required is to hand. Never encourage a dog to jump into or out of a bath in case of injury – always lift in. Do not leave unattended in case the dog panics.

Use collar restraint to attach the dog to the bath, leaving both the groomer's hands free. A nylon collar and lead is used, never a chain. If the dog panics or slips the nylon lead can be cut quickly, preventing injury.

The groomer should wear protective clothing and non-slip soles to shoes or boots, for safety. When using medicated and parasite shampoo, glove protection is required.

- Lift into the bath. Two people may be required to lift medium and large breeds.
- Stand dog on a non-slip mat.
- Regulate water temperature.
- Soak hindquarters first, using hands to force water through heavy coats.
- Continue soaking, moving last to the head and face, protecting the eyes from the water.
- Once the dog is soaked, introduce the shampoo, using hand and sponge. As before, start over the hindquarters and move towards the head, including abdomen, under the tail and between the foot pads but still protecting the eyes at all times.

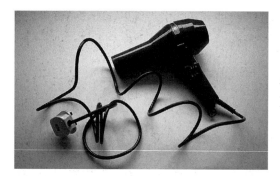

**Fig. 16.18** Hand-held dryer.

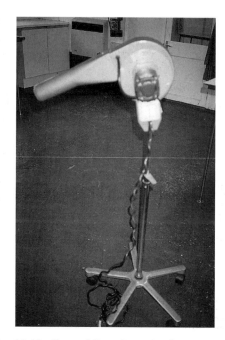

**Fig. 16.19** Type of floor dryer stand.

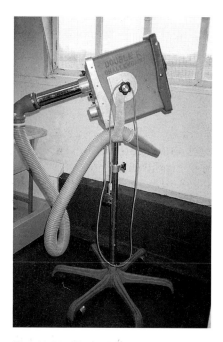

**Fig. 16.20** Type of floor dryer stand.

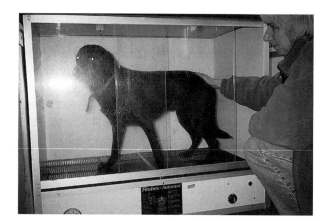

**Fig. 16.21** Cabinet dryer with false vented floor.

- Hold the head up to encourage water and shampoo to drain back along the spine while attending to the face and chin.
- Rinse off the shampoo.
- Repeat the application of shampoo (if medicated or parasite shampoo, leave in contact with the skin for correct amount of time).
- Rinse thoroughly.
- Squeeze water out of coat using hands or chamois-type cloth.
- Towel dry on a non-slip surface and place in a warm area to finish drying or dry using a dryer.
- Pat dry, never rub vigorously with long coats as this will create tangles.

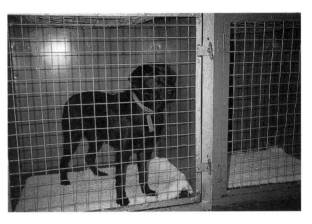

**Fig. 16.23**   In the holding kennel awaiting collection by owner.

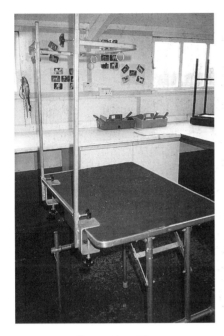

**Fig. 16.22**   Grooming table.

During the drying stage the coat can be brushed out. The object of using the dryer to dry some breeds is to get the coat as fluffy as possible. To achieve this, the coat is dried in sections, brushing constantly to straighten curls.

Finally, trim nails if necessary and clip hair between foot pads. Professional groomers would then proceed with the plucking, stripping, clipping and scissoring required by certain breeds, depending on coat type and requirements. This would be done on a grooming table (Fig. 16.22). The dog would then be transferred to the holding kennel to await collection by the owner (Fig. 16.23).

## Cats

Grooming provides the owner with the opportunity not only to condition the coat and skin but to:

- Clean any discharge and examine the eyes
- Clean ears and check for signs of infection, excess wax or ear mites
- Examine mouth and check teeth for build-up of tartar and for gum disease
- Examine and trim claws and clean claw bed of caked-on dirt
- Clean dirty coat
- Check for skin parasites

Grooming should begin from the time of weaning to accustom a kitten to short but daily coat care. As with the dog, this also becomes a bonding/playtime session between the owner and the animal. This attention is particularly important if the kitten is to be a show animal.

Cats spend a considerable part of every day in self-grooming. They have a specially adapted tongue with backward-facing barbs for the removal of dead hairs from the coat.

Grooming will:

- Remove dead hair
- Remove material from coat surface
- Stimulate skin and distribute secreted oils for coat condition
- Provide a feeling of well-being

Constant grooming in long-haired cats can cause health problems. During self-grooming the cat will swallow large quantities of saliva and wet hair, which forms *hair balls* or sausage-shaped plugs in the stomach. This ingested hair can cause an obstruction in the digestive tract.

In the event of loss of appetite, weight loss or constipation, contact a veterinary surgeon for advice.

## The coat

Selective breeding and genetic mutation have enhanced cats' coats or caused coat loss. The cat has a top coat of *guard hair* and an undercoat which consists of coarse, bristly *awn* hairs and soft downy hairs.

Examples of coat type are as follows:

- *Short hair*, e.g. British short hair, has short guard hairs with even shorter but slightly curly awn hairs as a sparse undercoat.
- *Long hair*, e.g. Persian, has extremely long guard hairs with a thick undercoat of downy hair which gives this breed its full, dense coat.
- *Curly coat*, e.g. Cornish Rex, has very short curly awn and downy hairs of the same length and no guard hairs at all.
- *Wire hair*, e.g. American wire hair, has short curly, even coiled guard hairs, down and awn.
- *Hairless*, e.g. Sphinx, which has a coat so sparse as to appear hairless but in fact has a covering of downy hairs on the legs, tail and face only.

The cat has three kinds of skin gland to care for its coat. Two types are sweat-producing glands, some located only on the pads of the feet, others over the entire body used to leave its scent and mark territory. Territory marking is seen when the cat rubs against objects. The third type of gland is the sebaceous gland near the hair follicles which secretes sebum to help waterproof the coat.

Moulting occurs in the spring and autumn, when the coat comes out in what seem like handfulls at a time. Long-haired coats moult all year round due to the constant room temperatures in which these cats tend to live. It is therefore essential that the long-coated breeds have owners who realise the necessity of daily grooming routines.

## Grooming notes

### Short coat

These cats are efficient self-groomers, with the normal-shaped head giving a slightly longer tongue than in the long-coated breeds. Two half-hour grooming sessions per week are ideal. In between, continue to condition the coat by stroking along the lie of the hair or polishing the coat using a piece of silk, velvet or chamois leather cloth.

Equipment required:

- Fine-toothed comb
- Soft bristle brush
- Rubber brush (see Fig. 16.7)
- Chamois cloth

### Long coat

With the shorter faces resulting in shorter tongues, these breeds tend to be less efficient groomers. Moulting all year round, the coat tends to mat. Grooming is needed daily, split into two half-hour sessions during the day to check for mats. Start with a normal comb to remove dead hair and then use a fine comb to fluff up the coat. A toothbrush is used to brush the face hair, keeping well clear of the eyes.

Equipment required:

- Wide-toothed and fine-toothed combs
- Slicker brush
- Bristle brush
- Toothbrush – medium bristle

### Curly coat

Should not be overgroomed as this could result in baldness. A soft brush with short bristles is sufficient for removal of dead coat. Groom twice weekly.

Equipment required:

- Soft bristle brush

*Wire coat*

These have a crimped, woolly coat which is coarse to the touch. Removal of the dead hair is essential but ensure that the curls spring untangled back into position. This is achieved by minimum brushing with a soft bristle brush and hand stroking at least twice weekly.

Equipment required:

- Soft bristle brush

*Hairless coat*

With hair only on extremities, skin conditioning is more essential. Do not brush these breeds. The skin needs daily sponging to remove *dander* (small scales from the hair and dried skin secretions). A sponge moistened with warm water wiped over the body daily or more frequently if required will remove the dander which, if left, could cause a skin allergy.

Equipment required:

- Sponge

## Bathing

Groom out all mats and hair contaminated with faeces. If these mats cannot be groomed out, it may be necessary to cut them off with scissors.

As with the dog, make sure all equipment is to hand before starting. A non-slip surface in the bath is essential in order to give the cat something to cling to. Unless bathing is a routine experience, cats can find it very traumatic so only bath if really necessary.

Two people are required, one to hold and reassure, one to bath.

- Fill the bath with about 10 cm of warm water into which the cat is lowered gently.
- A mixer hose and/or a sponge are used to soak the coat hair and apply the shampoo. Proceed with a thorough rinse and then wrap the cat in a towel.
- At all times, make sure water or shampoo never gets close to the eyes, ears or mouth.
- Wipe over the face with cotton wool moistened in warm water.
- Towel dry and keep in a warm area until fully dry.
- If the cat will tolerate it, use an electric dryer set only to warm and held at a safe distance.
- Once the coat is dry, comb out gently and brush.

Finish with the grooming of the coat hair.

- *Short hair* – start at the head and comb/brush towards the tail, including chest and abdomen. Then rub down with a chamois or nylon pad to polish the coat.
- *Long hair* – comb legs free of tangles then abdomen, flanks, back, chest and neck, then the tail section, fluffing out the coat hair by brushing the wrong way. Finally, using a toothbrush, groom the face hair.

When all grooming is complete, remove the dead hair from the combs and brushes, wash, disinfect and rinse before storing to prevent cross infection between grooming sessions or infecting another animal groomed with the same equipment.

### Warning

If the coat is dirtied by chemicals such as tar, creosote, paint or oil, remove as soon as possible to prevent absorption through the skin or self-grooming and ingestion of the chemical, which may be a poison. Never use chemicals to remove these substances. On a dry coat, use soft margarine, washing-up liquid or liquid paraffin to work the substance free of the hairs, then proceed with a bath and dry thoroughly. If the cat has self-groomed, contact a veterinary surgeon immediately for advice.

# Chapter 17
# Small Mammals

Small mammals may not be used to handling and can bite. Initial restraint should be firm but gentle to prevent injury (Fig. 17.1).

## General husbandry

### Housing

Cages, runs and pens need to be well made and of materials suitable to the species being housed. To prevent injury, housing should:

- Have no sharp edges
- Have no rough surfaces
- Be in good repair
- Be easy to clean
- Be escape proof
- Be large enough for free movement and exercise
- Be dry and well ventilated
- Be heated or cooled as required during the seasonal changes in environmental temperature
- Have a supply of electricity
- Have no direct sunlight into housing
- Not be subject to temperature extremes

### Health

A regular examination to determine health status or detect injury is required. If any animal is found to be diseased it is important to move it to isolation or quarantine areas.

Only purchase animals from a reputable and reliable source. It is easy to introduce disease to an animal collection which can be hard to treat and eliminate.

To maintain health:

- Clean housing thoroughly
- Move any sick animal to isolation

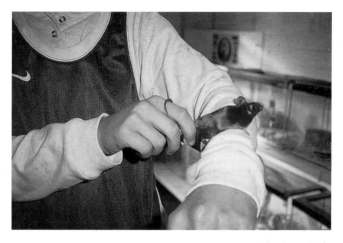

**Fig. 17.1**  Gentle restraint, allowing the mouse to explore without escaping.

- Apply high levels of hygiene to all equipment
- Have a good air flow through the housing to prevent breathing problems and airborne diseases
- House different species separately where possible
- Change bedding several times a week

## *Nutrition*

The needs of each species of animal have been well documented. However, there are general guidelines.

- Feed only fresh and clean leafy foods.
- Check the feed container is in date, has not been broken open or damaged and is not contaminated.
- Feed must provide all nutrients necessary for full health.
- Water is fresh and always available.
- Water containers/feeders are regularly cleaned.
- Food is stored in closed containers at room temperature and kept dry.

# Rabbits

## *Anatomical facts*

### *Eyes*

Rabbits have a wide field of vision, 190° for each eye. Dilation of the pupil means their night vision is about 7–8 times more effective than that of humans.

### Ears

Have a good blood supply and assist with body heat regulation and sound gathering.

### Teeth

Are open rooted, continuing to grow throughout life. If the correct foods and environment are provided, the teeth are continually worn down, which is essential for health.

### Thoracic cavity

This is small, allowing for a large abdomen, which houses a lengthy intestinal tract with a large caecum.

### Skeleton

Light, delicate bones, covered with powerful muscle system, especially to the hind legs. This can mean the limbs and spine are prone to fracture, if handled carelessly.

### Scent glands

Located in the anal region for marking of territory.

### Lifespan

Five to six years or more.

## Housing

There are many texts providing plans and layouts for both inside and outside housing. They also provide construction details for housing and runs and safe materials to use. Rabbits and guinea pigs can be kept together (Fig. 17.2).

Housing should:

- Protect from extremes of heat and cold. The preferred temperature is 12–20°C
- Be well constructed from good-quality materials. If materials have been treated, check the chemicals used are non-toxic
- Be the correct size, with separate compartments for living and sleeping
- Protect from predators by being raised and fitted with a sturdy catch/lock system

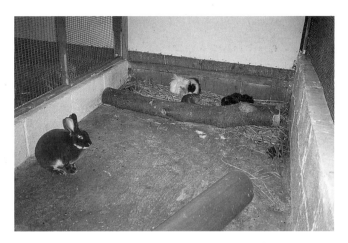

**Fig. 17.2**    Example of group housing of rabbit and guinea pig.

- Contain materials for gnawing to reduce the teeth length. A supply of bark-covered logs from non-toxic trees (i.e. fruit trees) should be regularly changed
- Include a portable outdoor 'summer' run for natural grazing
- Provide good ventilation
- Be easy to clean. Remove soiled bedding at least twice weekly. Disinfect at least monthly to remove the scale and odour from housing

### Food and water

Many rabbits are fed on commercially produced pelleted foods which may contain anticoccidial agents which could be harmful to some species. Check the packaging if rabbits and guinea pigs feed together as these additives would be harmful to the guinea pig.

Rabbits are herbivores so the main diet should consist of roughage: good-quality hay or grass, supplemented by cereals, leafy greens and vegetables. Select vegetables and greens carefully. Do not feed if any of the following are suspected or present:

- Greens are not fresh picked.
- Mould is visible.
- The feed is frozen or unwashed.
- It has been sprayed with chemicals or weedkillers.
- The plant may be poisonous to some species of animal.

Rabbits naturally eats their own faecal pellets (*coprophagia*), usually in the early morning with a supplied diet. The rabbit passes two types of faecal pellet:

(1)  *Dry pellets* – waste faecal materials.
(2)  *Moist pellets* – are eaten directly from the anus. These *caecal pellets* are mucus covered and stick together and are passed twice through the digestive system for maximum extraction of nutrient material.

Fresh water must be available at all times, from a water bottle and spout or a drinking bowl.

# Guinea pigs

## *Anatomical facts*

### Teeth

Are open rooted, continuing to grow throughout the guinea pig's lifetime.

### Tail

Born without a tail.

### Scent glands

Sebaceous glands are located on the rump and used to mark territory.

### Pelvis

The pubic symphysis (floor of the pelvic joint) will separate under the influence of hormones during parturition, in order to allow the newborn passage through the birth canal. Newborn guinea pigs are referred to as *precocious*, meaning that within a few hours of birth they are self-sufficient, eating and drinking from feeding dishes. They are born with a complete coat, eyes and ears open and with a set of teeth in place.

### Lifespan

Four to five years.

## *Housing*

Guinea pigs are sociable and can be housed as a colony. A single animal is often housed with another species such as a rabbit.
Housing should:

- Protect from extremes of temperature, similar to the rabbit.
- Protect the animal from getting wet.

- Be well constructed from good-quality materials which have not been treated with any toxic chemicals.
- Be the correct size; a rabbit housing can accommodate 2–3 guinea pigs.
- Provide good air flow and ventilation.
- Have a summer run for natural grazing.
- Be easy to clean. Guinea pigs tend not to toilet in one area so more frequent cleaning is required than for the rabbit. If feeding and water bowls are used, these need daily washing as they tend to be fouled.

### Food and water

Guinea pigs often chew feed and water containers. Choose a suitable indestructible material.

Guinea pigs are herbivores and spend most waking hours grazing if allowed. By nature, guinea pigs dislike any change to their routines so watch for correct use of water feeders, if any changes have been made to equipment.

Commercially available pelleted guinea pig feed can be used. If any other prepared diet is used, then it is essential to supplement vitamin C as ascorbic acid in the diet for skin and coat condition. Some rabbit diets may also contain levels of vitamin D that are too high for the guinea pig. Read the packaging and ask the supplier for advice. Supply good-quality roughage like hay or cut grass. Supplement pelleted food with fresh vegetables and fruit. Always provide fresh drinking water.

## Mice

### Anatomical facts

#### Teeth

Are open rooted and continue to grow (incisor teeth only).

#### Lifespan

Eighteen months to three years.

### Housing

It is important that mice housing is environmentally enriched with tubes, ropes, exercise wheels and compartments. All will enable the mouse to exercise and keep busy for health and fitness.

Mice may be housed in small groups or alone. They are usually active throughout the day with rest periods.

Housing should:

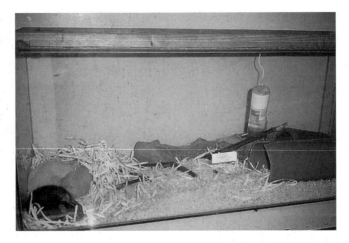

**Fig. 17.3** Housing with plenty of compartments.

- Be escape proof
- Be kept inside
- Have no direct sunlight
- Be cleaned at least twice a week to reduce odour and accumulation of urine and faeces
- Be dry and easy to clean
- Contain activities (Fig. 17.3)

### Food and water

Mice are omnivores. Diets in pellet form are available. Mice require some animal-based protein in their diet which the commercial foods will provide. They benefit from pieces of fruit and vegetable in small quantities.

Remove any uneaten food materials.

Water must be provided at all times, via a water bottle and sipper tube.

## Rats

### Anatomical facts

#### Teeth

Rats have open-rooted incisor teeth which continue to grow.

#### Long bones

Ossify in the second year of life.

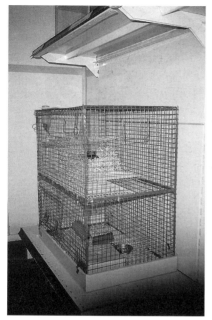

**Fig. 17.4** Type of housing with two levels for a rat.

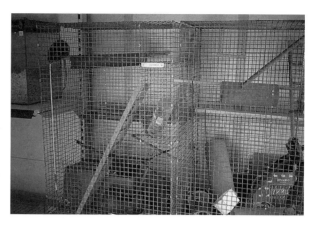

**Fig. 17.5** Close-up view of a two-level house.

### Digestive tract

Rats have a divided stomach, large caecum and no gall bladder.

### Lifespan

Two and a half to $3\frac{1}{2}$ years.

## Housing

Rats will live in small groups or alone but do need plenty of space for activity. They can become attached to their owners, are quick to learn and easy to train. Rats will burrow given the opportunity and can be nocturnal.

Housing should:

- Provide enough space for sleeping and activity areas
- Be inside but not in direct sunlight
- Be interesting with different levels (Figs 17.4 and 17.5), but easy to clean
- Be cleaned 2–3 times per week to reduce odour, urine and faeces
- Be gnaw proof and made of materials not treated with toxic chemicals

### *Food and water*

Rats are omnivores. They do not eat strange or new foods readily. As for mice, diets can be bought in pellet form. Check packaging for a high protein content. The rat will also eat scraps from the table, fruit and some vegetables. Provide with fresh water using bottle and sipper tube to prevent contamination.

## Hamsters

### *Anatomical facts*

*Teeth*

Incisors are open rooted.

*Mouth*

Has large cheek pouches, reaching almost to the scapula area of the shoulder, used to transport food or temporarily store it.

*Scent glands*

Situated in the flank region and used to mark territory, these are seen as darker patches of skin and are also known as *flank glands*.

*Lifespan*

One and a half to two years.

### *Housing*

Hamsters are naturally solitary animals, tending to fight in group situations. They are nocturnal but if disturbed from sleep, will bite. When awake, they have a lot of energy. Hamsters in the wild will dig tunnels close to the surface. If the temperature of their environment drops below 5°C they may hibernate for survival.

They chew soft metals, plastic and wood. Care with bedding and activity equipment is necessary as the hamster will chew and pouch any material, which may in turn cause pouch infections.

Housing should:

* Have only safe bedding materials such as peat or wood shavings as a base, covered with untreated paper or cardboard for shredding and nesting
* Be kept inside
* Not be in direct sunlight

- Be well constructed and gnaw proof
- Be cleaned at least 2–3 times a week
- Provide exercise equipment such as a wheel, tunnels, ladders and plenty of safe materials for shredding

### Food and water

The hamster is an omnivore, therefore a commercially produced 'hamster mix' food can be used. The diet should contain some animal protein. Vegetables and fruit will help to improve health status.

Provide fresh drinking water using a water bottle and sipper tube.

# Gerbils

### Anatomical facts

#### Scent glands

Situated on the abdomen, these glands are used for identification and marking of territory.

#### Adrenal glands

Hormones from these endocrine glands assist the gerbil's ability to conserve water in adverse conditions.

#### Hind legs

Longer than front legs for escape from predators.

#### Tail

Used for balance and turning. If grasped away from its base, the tail skin will slough to allow escape.

#### Lifespan

Three to four years.

### Housing

Gerbils are social animals and will live in groups, but can be aggressive to any newcomer. They are active during daylight hours (*diurnal*). As pets, they are easy to handle, clean and friendly.

Gerbils are adapted to live in extremes of temperature, from 43°C to below freezing. The gerbil is a burrowing animal, creating elaborate tunnel systems and entrances. The burrowing material, peat, hay or wood shavings, needs to be dampened and impacted at the base of the housing to allow this tunnel building.

The ideal housing is a fish tank or glass-sided tank, with a mesh lid. Allow enough room between the lid and the tunnel material for aboveground or surface activity.

Housing should:

- Be escape proof
- Contain only non-toxic materials, as gerbils will gnaw anything in their environment
- Be in a warm environment; 18–29°C is ideal
- Be a gerbilarium – an enclosure not less than a metre long, prepared with layers of dampened peat and straw
- Be washed, disinfected and rinsed monthly
- Have good light levels in the daytime, to encourage activity

Gerbils produce only a few drops of urine and faecal pellets are dry and odourless so bedding only needs to be changed about every 2–4 weeks, unless it is particularly dirty.

## Food and water

The gerbil is an omnivore but its diet includes grain, seeds and greens. Intake of sunflower seeds should be restricted as these are too rich in fat and calcium which can lead to dietary imbalance and ill health. Animal protein source may be provided by a commercial gerbil food or be supplemented via table scraps or boiled egg.

The gerbil will hoard food in a larder area of its housing. Water must be supplied in bottles with sipper tubes and these can be attached to the side of the tank or the lid. The water should be supplied fresh daily.

# Section 3
# Nursing

# Chapter 18
# First Aid and Nursing

## First aid

This is the emergency care and treatment of an animal with sudden illness or injury, before medical and surgical care (veterinary treatment) can be commenced. The main objectives at this time are to:

- Keep the animal alive
- Make it comfortable
- Assist in pain control
- Prevent its condition getting worse

Different situations require different approaches. Some situations will allow plenty of time to attend to injuries or problems and never be life threatening. Other situations are so severe the animal will die if urgent and skilled emergency care is not available.

First aid, being only the initial actions of someone attending or witnessing an accident, is very limited. It does not involve diagnosis or medical treatment of injuries but is designed to preserve life and temporarily prevent a condition getting worse if possible. It should allow time to get the animal to a veterinary surgeon who can diagnose the full extent of the condition, which is not always obvious at first.

## Evaluating situations

### Very severe

Must act immediately or the animal will die.

- The heart has stopped (*cardiopulmonary arrest*)
- Breathing is obstructed due to an object in the air passages
- Breathing has stopped
- Bleeding from a main artery or vein
- Acute allergic reaction to insect sting or other substance

### Severe

Must act within one hour or the animal may die.

- Deep cuts and considerable blood loss
- Established shock
- Head injuries
- Breathing difficulties

### Serious

Must act within 4–5 hours or more serious problems will develop that could be life threatening.

- Bone fractures that puncture through the skin (*compound fractures*)
- Spinal injuries
- Early stages of shock
- Difficulties in giving birth (*dystocia*)

### Major

Must act within 24 hours to prevent further damage.

- Fractures with no skin injury (*simple fractures*)
- Prolonged vomiting and diarrhoea
- Foreign bodies in the eyes or ears

## Initial management

(1) *Assess the situation and keep calm* – briefly examine the animal and note obvious injuries.
(2) *Contact the veterinary practice* – for advice and to let them know you are coming.
(3) *Ensure your own safety* – make sure the animal is properly restrained before handling and lifting, so that no one is bitten.
(4) *Stop and cover any obvious bleeding* – use sterile dressings if possible to prevent further contamination.
(5) *Make sure the animal is able to breathe* – if the airway is obstructed, clear it.
(6) *Treat for shock* – by maintaining the body temperature.

## Handling and transport

If the animal's life is in danger, then it must be moved. Injured animals are usually in pain, shocked and frightened and may attack anyone who tries to approach or handle them.

In order to protect both the handler and the animal from further harm or injury, great care is needed at this time.

- Slow deliberate movements are essential.
- A calm, soothing voice will help.
- Handle the animal as little as possible.
- Muzzle if necessary and only if the animal has no breathing difficulties.
- Transport to the surgery.

Before moving the animal, quickly assess the condition. This is referred to as *initial help* and if this can be started as soon as possible, the chances of survival are greatly improved. The initial assessment and help given must then be reported to the veterinary staff on arrival at the surgery, in order to reduce delay in treatment.

Checks to make are as follows:

- *Airway* – to ensure it is not obstructed; if it is, then clear it.
- *Breathing* – to make sure this is possible and assist with artificial respiration if required.
- *Heart and pulse* – check the beat, its rate and strength and record the information. If the heart has stopped, then proceed with heart massage (see p. 195).

Species consideration is important when considering handling. The method for moving an injured dog will vary from the method used for horses, cattle or birds.

### Small dogs, cats, rabbits and smaller pets

Transport in a pet carrier or in a cat-sized basket, making sure there are plenty of breathing holes. A lot of owners now own a cat cage, which is ideal for many species, provided there is plenty of space to stretch out (Fig. 18.1) or can be held in the owner's arms depending at the injury (Fig. 18.2).

### Medium-sized dogs

If they only have minor injuries then they may be encouraged to walk slowly. If they are not able to walk, then pick them up with one arm around the front of the forelegs and one around the hind legs (providing this is not contraindicated by the injuries), lift and hold against your body, with the legs hanging downward (Figs 18.3, 18.4).

### Large breeds of dog or similar

These should only be lifted by more than one person, one supporting the head and chest and another supporting abdomen and hindquarters. If the dog is too

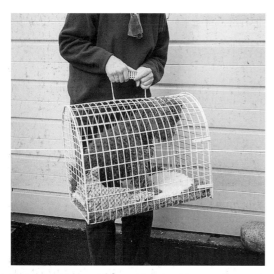

**Fig. 18.1**   Carrier cage for a small dog or cat.

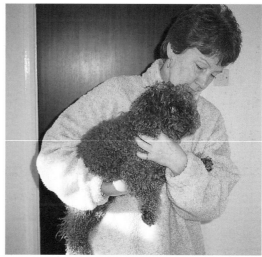

**Fig. 18.2**   Small dog held in arms.

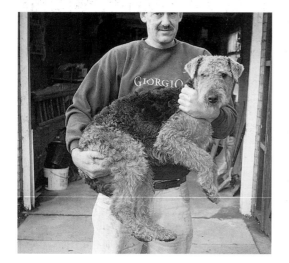

**Fig. 18.3**   × Wrong – the arm on the neck is too high.

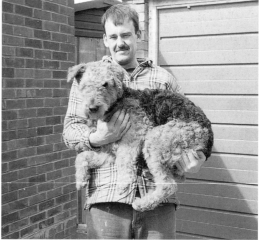

**Fig. 18.4**   ✓ Right – the arm has been lowered and will not now obstruct breathing.

large for lifting, then with two or more handlers use a stretcher or blanket lift (Fig. 18.5). Pull the animal onto the blanket lying on its side and lift using the corners of the blanket or, if not enough handlers are available, simply drag the blanket, providing the surface is smooth. This blanket technique is also used for smaller animals with spinal injuries (Fig. 18.6).

Whatever the size of the injured animal always lift in the correct manner; bend your knees before lifting rather than bending from the waist. The handler's own back is less at risk but if in doubt, get more help (Fig. 18.7).

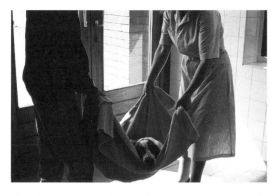

**Fig. 18.5** Blanket lift requires two or more people for a large dog.

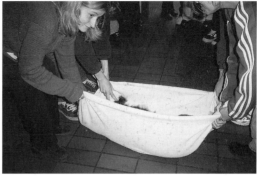

**Fig. 18.6** Blanket lift for a smaller dog with spinal injuries.

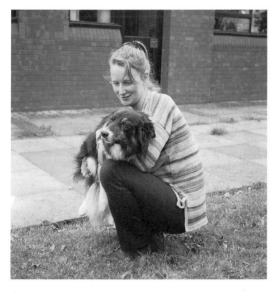

**Fig. 18.7** Lift with straight back and bent knees to prevent handler back strain injury.

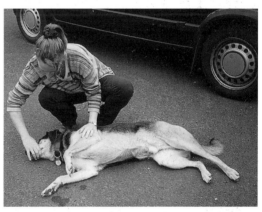

**Fig. 18.8** Recovery position for an injured animal, keeping the airway straight.

## Recovery position

As in human first aid, in animal first aid there is a *recovery position* in which to place the animal to ensure breathing is assisted and the heart is exposed for emergency procedures, if required (Fig. 18.8).

- Lie the animal on its right side.
- Straighten head and neck.
- Tongue is pulled forward and behind the canine tooth (to one side of the mouth).

- Remove any collar or harness.
- Check the heart and pulse regularly.

Other checks to make and record at this time include the following.
- Any signs of *bleeding* from the animal's surface or from a body opening like the mouth, rectum, vulva, prepuce or ears.
- *Colour* is checked by looking at the lining of the lower eyelid and the mucous membrane of the mouth and gums.

---

**Colour of mucous membranes**

- *Pale* – indicating shock or serious bleeding (internal or external).
- *Blue* – also referred to as *cyanotic*, indicates lack of oxygen to the tissue cells.
- *Yellow* – also referred to as *jaundice*, can be caused by an excess of bile pigment in the bloodstream and usually involves the liver in some way.
- *Red/congested* – indicates overoxygenation after exercise, in heat stroke cases or fever conditions.

---

- The *capillary refill time* is checked. The upper lip is lifted and the gum over the top canine tooth is pressed. This squeezes the blood out of the surface capillaries, causing the area to go temporarily white. The refill time is the time it takes to become the normal pink colour again as the capillaries refill, usually 1–1½ seconds. Any time longer than that is considered 'slow' and may indicate a degree of shock.
- *Rate and quality of the pulse*. This is taken in the groin area of the hind leg on the femoral artery. This artery is exposed over the femur bone at this point, allowing the pulse to be taken. Another artery that may be used is the sublingual, under the animal's tongue, but this is only used in unconscious animals. *Rate* refers to the speed of the pulse which is a reflection of the heart beat. The pulse should be taken for a full minute for a true recording. The *quality* of the pulse refers to qualities such as strong, thready, weak or normal. In order to describe this, the handler must have some experience of pulse taking.
- *Breathing rate* is recorded describing whether it is normal, slow, fast or shallow.
- *Body temperature* is taken if a thermometer is available. If not, then feel the extremities of the body like the feet and tail end. If the temperature is lower than it should be, the handler will feel this because most animals (mammals and birds) have a body temperature higher than humans.
- Record its *level of consciousness*; in other words, can the animal respond to stimuli like its name, a noise or sudden movement.
- Record any *unusual odour* on the animal's body, whether it comes from the animal's mouth, anus or coat.

# Life-saving techniques

(1)   The heart has stopped – *cardiac arrest*.
(2)   The breathing has stopped – *respiratory arrest*.

The two above situations are jointly referred to as *cardiopulmonary arrest* (*pulmonary* refers to the vessels that take blood to the lungs and back to the heart).

The object of cardiopulmonary resuscitation is to restore heart and lung action and to prevent irreversible brain damage which would happen if the tissues were deprived of oxygen for any length of time. Damage to body cells is thought to occur after 3–4 minutes following cardiac arrest. Therefore, being adequately prepared is the most important step in the management of these emergencies and recognising that time is short if permanent damage to body tissues is to be avoided.

## Cardiac compression (heart massage)

### Small dogs or cats or other small animals

- Place in recovery position (on its right side, head and neck extended and tongue pulled forwards).
- Take hold of its chest between the thumb and fingers of the same hand, over the heart and just behind the elbows.
- Support the body of the animal with the other hand on the lumbar spine area.
- At all times, keep the head and neck in a straight line to assist breathing.
- Squeeze the thumb and fingers of the hand over the heart together; this will compress the chest wall and the heart, which is squeezed between the ribs.
- Repeat this action approximately 120 times per minute.
- Watch for the heart contractions restarting.

### Medium-sized dogs and other species

- Place in recovery position.
- Put the heel of one hand on the top of the chest, just behind the elbow and over the heart (Figs 18.9, 18.10).
- Place the other hand either on top of the first hand or under the animal to support the heart as it is compressed.
- Press down onto the chest with firm, sharp movements.
- Repeat this action about 80–100 times per minute.
- Watch for the heart contractions restarting.

### Large, barrel-chested or fat dogs and other species

- Place on its back, with its head slightly lower than its body if possible.
- Put the heel of one hand on the abdominal end of the sternum (breast bone).

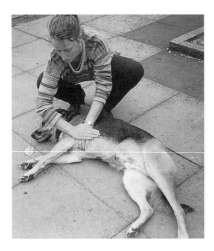

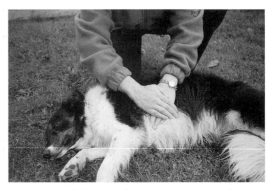

**Fig. 18.10** Same hand position, behind the elbow, over the heart.

**Fig. 18.9** Position for hands when doing cardiac massage.

- Place the other hand on top of the first.
- Press firmly onto the chest, pushing the hands forwards towards the head of the animal.
- Press down in this way 80–100 times per minute.
- Keep the head and neck straight during the procedure, at all times.
- Watch for the heart restarting.

With all animals, stop at 20-second intervals to check for heart beat or pulse, then continue.

## Respiratory arrest

Whatever the cause, if the breathing has stopped then it must urgently be restarted. Resuscitation methods do include the use of drugs which stimulate the heart and the breathing but these are only administered by a veterinary surgeon and therefore are not a first aid procedure.

There are two methods for restarting the breathing:

(1)   Artificial respiration – manual method
(2)   Mouth-to-nose technique

### Artificial respiration

- Place in recovery position.
- Clear airway of any blocking material.
- Place a hand over the ribs, behind the shoulder bone (Fig. 18.11).
- Compress the chest with a sharp downward movement.

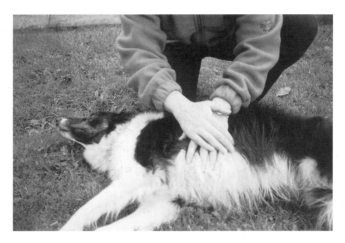

**Fig. 18.11**   For artificial respiration compression, hands are placed over the chest.

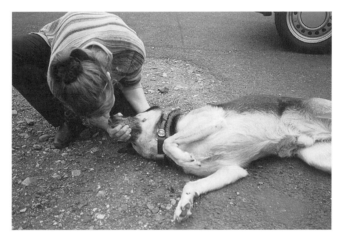

**Fig. 18.12**   Mouth-to-nose resuscitation with the airway kept straight and mouth held shut. The operator breaths down the nose.

- Allow the chest to expand and then repeat the downward movement.
- Repeat approximately every 3–5 seconds, until breathing restarts.
- Keep head and neck straight at all times to maintain airway.

*Mouth-to-nose technique*

- Place in recovery position.
- Clear the airway.
- Place a tissue or thin cloth over the animal's nose (for personal safety).
- Hold the animal's neck straight at all times.
- Keep its mouth closed by holding upper and lower jaws together.
- Breathe down its nose to inflate the lungs (Fig. 18.12).

- Repeat this inflation of the lungs at 3–5-second intervals.
- Watch for the breathing restarting.

This technique provides the animal with the unused oxygen in the handler's breath and their exhaled carbon dioxide, which helps to stimulate the breathing or gasp reflex in the animal.

## Poisons

A poison or toxin is any substance which, on entry to the body in sufficient amounts, has a harmful effect on the individual. Poisons can gain entry to the body by various means.

- By mouth
- Via the lungs
- Absorbed through the skin surface
- Through a cut

Animals can be poisoned by a multitude of potentially toxic substances, many of which are ordinary household products. The source may be poisonous plants or toxic chemicals used or stored near the animal in the kitchen or utility room where a dog or cat may have its bed. Such poisons would include:

- Pesticides for the garden like slug bait, Path Clear, moss killer etc.
- Rodent killers like warfarin poison
- Paint and cleaning solutions for brushes
- Disinfectants like bleach and toilet cleaners
- Drugs like aspirin, blood pressure tablets and sleeping tablets

Very few poisons produce distinctive signs. Most cause non-specific signs such as the following:

- Becoming aggressive, excited or depressed
- Unsteady on its feet
- Salivating, vomiting and/or having diarrhoea
- Abdominal pain and fitting-type episodes
- Pale, with lowered body temperature
- Slow capillary refill time

The owner knows best what is normal and what is unusual in their pet so record all reported information and get in touch with the veterinary surgeon as soon as possible for advice on what to do next. If the owner knows the chemical involved and has the container or packet, take that to the veterinary surgeon too. Unless instructed to make the animal sick, do not attempt to do so as this may cause more harm.

Until the veterinary surgeon takes over:

- Place in recovery position
- Support for any breathing problems
- Keep warm to reduce shock
- Record pulse and heart rate
- Comfort and do not leave unattended

Get to the veterinary surgeon as soon as possible.


## Insect stings

These are usually more painful than harmful. However, it is possible that an animal may have an allergic reaction to the insect venom or that the sting is near the airway and could obstruct breathing.

If the venom sac is imbedded in the skin, never squeeze it as this may inject more venom into the animal. Remove carefully if possible or leave it in place for the veterinary surgeon to remove in the safety of the practice.

*Wasp stings* are alkaline. Treatment is therefore with an acid solution like household vinegar in the form of a pad or compress.

*Bee stings* are acid. Treatment is therefore with an alkali such as bicarbonate of soda mixed with water and soaked into a pad or compress.

Treatment aims to neutralise the situation. It is not always possible to know which insect is involved unless someone has seen it happen. If this is the case, then apply a cold compress or face flannel filled with ice cubes to the area to reduce the swelling and give some pain control.


## Bleeding or haemorrhage

Bleeding or *haemorrhage* is the escape of blood from damaged blood vessels and can cause serious problems. Bleeding heavily can decrease the circulating blood volume enough to cause shock. Bleeding that is less heavy may still cause the tissue cells to be deprived of oxygen, which could be permanently damaging. Even small losses of blood can delay wound healing and contribute to development of an infection. Therefore any loss potentially puts the animal at risk.

Bleeding is not always obvious; it may be *internal*, especially after a road traffic accident, so watch for the general signs:

- Colour is pale
- Attitude is dull or listless
- Appears thirsty
- The pulse and breathing rate are fast and may appear feeble
- Feet and tail are cold to touch
- Body temperature is subnormal
- Capillary refill time is slow

If blood loss is severe then signs include those of blood loss to vital organs, such as the following:

- Animal becomes restless and will not settle
- It has difficulty breathing
- May have fitting-type episode
- Unable to stand and becomes unconscious

For reporting purposes, the following information is useful to the veterinary surgeon:

- What type of blood vessel is damaged
- Where on the body the injury is
- When the bleeding started
- Is the bleeding internal or surface?
- Treatments carried out so far

---

**Which blood vessel is damaged?**

- *Artery* – blood is bright red (oxygenated) in colour and comes out as spurts, which are synchronised with the heart beat.
- *Vein* – blood is dark red (deoxygenated) in colour and is a steady flow.
- *Capillary* – is bright red and seen as a steady ooze.

---

## Methods of arresting bleeding

The following methods are only for temporary application until the veterinary surgeon takes over.

### Digital (finger) pressure

Used on a surface wound by pressing a sterile or clean pad of absorbent material onto the area to control the blood loss. Care must be used with this method in case there is a piece of metal, glass or wood imbedded in the wound tissues;

pressing on this would push it deeper, where it would be harder to locate or may cause damage to internal structures.

This method can be used for about 5–15 minutes before tissues beyond must receive a reviving flow. Then pressure can be re-established.

### Pressure points

In several locations around the body, major arteries are near the body surface. These tend to supply the extremities like limbs and tail. Where they cross a bone, pressure can slow or even stop the supply reaching an area beyond. If the wound is on the extremity, these points can be used as a temporary measure.

- *Forelimbs* – the pressure is put on the inside or medial elbow area to slow the brachial artery flow.
- *Hind limbs* – the pressure is put on the same site used for pulse taking, in the groin area on the femur, to slow the femoral artery flow.
- *Tail* – the pressure is applied to the ventral or underside of the base of the tail to slow the coccygeal artery flow.

These locations can be used for about 5–10 minutes, before allowing the blood to flow to restore distant tissues.

### Pressure bandages

These may be used initially or after one or both of the above methods have been used to establish the extent of the injury.

Pressure bandages can only be applied to extremities, like limbs and tail. They are applied tightly to constrict and slow the surface vessels supplying the area, thus limiting blood loss.

Plenty of padding material is applied over the dressing on the wound and is then tightly bandaged in place. If blood seeps through, then more padding is applied and bandaged in place.

This is still only a temporary measure to be used before arriving at the veterinary surgery and will give about one hour of time before the tissues must be released from the tight bandage and flow restored.

## Shock

Shock is a term used to describe a very complex and potentially fatal clinical syndrome which always involves insufficient blood to the tissues, resulting in lack of oxygen to the cells. Lack of oxygen to the cells is called *tissue hypoxia* and this can be fatal if not corrected.

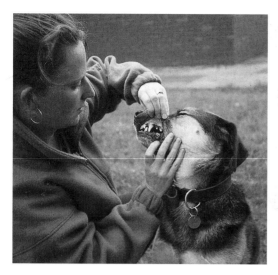

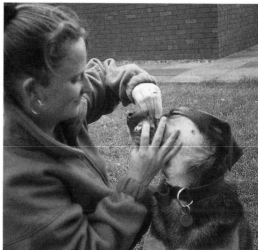

**Fig. 18.13**  Mucous membrane colour check.       **Fig. 18.14**  Capillary refill time check.

When blood is lost from the body, the body tries to compensate by redistributing blood to vital structures like the brain and heart at the expense of other organs like kidneys, skin, intestines and muscles. Organs can be severely damaged by the resulting tissue hypoxia.

The causes of shock vary but some examples are:

- Blood loss from damaged vessels
- Trauma injuries to tissues from a road traffic accident
- Pain due to injury or surgical procedures
- Heart problems that interfere with the normal pumping action of the heart
- Infections which cause blood to 'pool out' in the capillary beds, by affecting the walls of the blood vessels

The *signs of shock* include:

- Pale colour (Fig. 18.13)
- Cold extremities
- Weak or slipping into unconscious state
- Increase in the heart rate and breathing
- Slow capillary refill time of longer than two seconds (Fig. 18.14)

Until the animal can be treated by a veterinary surgeon, the handler must start the preventive shock procedure. Maintaining body temperature is probably the single most useful thing that can be done. If the body is not allowed to shut down the peripheral vessels to the limbs and tail, shock will be at least delayed and possibly even prevented.

Shock takes three forms:

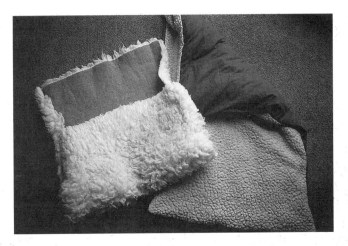

**Fig. 18.15**   Bedding types.

(1)   *Impending* – it is expected to happen, bearing in mind the events or injuries.
(2)   *Established* – it is in place and the animal must have urgent medical treatment involving whole blood transfusions or use of plasma expanders.
(3)   *Irreversible* – treatment is unlikely to save the animal's life as systems are too damaged.

Treatment is aimed at not allowing shock to move beyond the impending stage. To achieve this:

- Maintain body temperature by wrapping in blankets or towels (Fig. 18.15) and keep massaging or rubbing the extremities to stimulate the blood flow. Never use artificial heat as the temperature may get too high.
- Position the head slightly lower than the body to encourage the blood flow to the brain.
- Stop any further blood loss.
- Assist the animal to breathe by placing in the recovery position and give artificial respiration if breathing stops.
- Record the pulse.
- Get to the veterinary surgery as soon as possible.

## Bone fractures

A fracture refers to a crack in the surface of a bone or a complete break in a bone structure. The objectives of first aid for fractures are to prevent the situation getting worse and make the animal comfortable for transportation to the veterinary surgery.

The causes of bone fracture are varied and include:

- Road traffic accidents
- The animal landing badly after jumping
- Muscles contracting to break small bones in the legs of, particularly, racing dogs or horses
- Bone disease which has weakened the bone structure

---

**Types of fracture**

- *Simple* – bone is broken but there is no connecting skin injury (Fig. 18.16).
- *Compound* – bone is broken and there is a wound connecting to the skin or the bone is protruding through the skin. A badly handled simple fracture can become a compound.

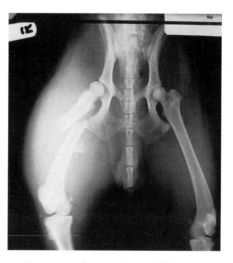

**Fig. 18.16**    X-ray shows fractured right femur and extent of tissue swelling.

---

The signs indicating a fracture include:

- Loss of use of affected limb, will not bear weight
- Pain on handling or will not allow handling
- Unusual position or shape to the limb
- Swelling and bruising
- Unusual movement of the limb

The best treatment for fractured bones is to get to the veterinary surgery quickly but taking care to cause no further injuries by careless handling. Some fractures are also complicated by damage to surrounding tissues like blood vessels, nerves or organs.

Depending on the fracture, first aid aims to:

* Stop any bleeding.
* Clean and cover any wounds.
* Immobilise the fracture site. This is only possible if the joint above and below the site can be immobilised by a splint. If splinting is possible, always apply the splint to the limb in the position in which it is found. For example, if the foot and carpals of the foreleg are now positioned sideways instead of facing front, do not correct the position – splint it.

Materials which can be used for splinting include:

* Rolled-up magazine or newspaper
* A ruler or piece of wood
* Cardboard
* A matchstick

If a splint is not possible then:

* Confine on plenty of bedding
* Comfort and do not leave unattended
* Treat for shock
* Get to the veterinary surgery

---

**What can be splinted?**

* *Forelimb* – from elbow to toes (*phalanges*).
* *Hind limb* – from stifle to toes.
* *Tail.*

---

# Wounds

A wound is damage to the continuous structure of any tissue in the body.

## Healing of a wound

### First-intention healing

Takes place in wounds that:

- Are not contaminated with grit, soil and micro-organisms
- Have cleancut edges that can be held together
- Have been cleaned within one hour of injury

In this type of healing, the edges rejoin by ten days postinjury.

### Second-intention healing or granulation

Takes place in wounds that:

- Are contaminated with grit, soil and micro-organisms
- Have jagged edges and possibly sections of skin missing
- Have not been cleaned within two hours of injury
- Have edges that gape open
- Become infected

This type of healing can take weeks to months.

## Types of wound

Wounds are described as being open or closed. The *closed* wound is one which does not penetrate the whole thickness of the skin as a structure, such as bruises or blood blisters (*haematoma*) or pockets of blood from a small damaged blood vessel. Treatment of these injuries involves use of a cold compress, such as ice cubes held in a face flannel, immediately postinjury to reduce the swelling of local tissues and help control pain. This treatment is only useful immediately postinjury.

*Open* wounds are those with damage to surface tissue and some bleeding. They are named according to the manner of the damage and whether or not tissue is missing.

- *Incised* – these have cleancut edges, are painful due to surface nerve ending damage and tend to bleed freely. Caused by sharp-edged materials like glass, metal or knife blade.
- *Lacerated* – these have very jagged flaps of skin and sometimes skin sections are missing (*avulsed*). However, because tissue is torn and stretched, they are less painful than incised wounds and do not bleed much. Caused by bite injuries, barbed wire or road traffic accident.

- *Puncture* – these wounds have a long narrow track deep into the tissues with only a small skin entry scab over the track. The scab holds any microbes in the track. The wound is caused by sharp pointed objects like teeth, in bite wounds, nails and thorns. These will all be contaminated with microbes, which are then left in the damage track to multiply, causing a local infection to develop. This local infection is held in the track area and, as it increases in size, is called an *abscess*. These are very painful, often causing loss of limb function.
- *Abrasions* – these have torn, ragged skin edges, with many contaminants embedded in the damaged areas. They are caused by a glancing blow or by being dragged along the ground briefly in a road traffic accident. The tissues tend to be torn and the damage only in the surface layers of the skin, so there is not much bleeding.

### Wound care

The sooner an open wound is cleaned using a water-based antiseptic solution, the more chance there is that infection will not develop. Solutions used for wound cleaning must not cause any further inflammation or damage to the wound and therefore should not contain any detergent.

If micro-organisms in the wound are prevented from multiplying, it could mean the difference between the wound healing within ten days (*first intention*) and the delayed healing of the second-intention or granulation method.

Solutions to use:

- Tap water
- 0.9% sodium chloride from a drip bag

Once cleaned, always cover the wound to prevent contamination and the animal aggravating the area further.

## Eye injuries

Any animal with eye injuries will be sight impaired and in pain. It is very important to approach slowly and talk to the animal so that it is warned of your approach. The animal will be frightened and could injure the handler unless precautions are observed and correct handling techniques used.

The types of injury seen include the following.

### Chemicals

These can cause serious injury to the eye structures. Always irrigate as soon as possible using tap water to remove any chemical. Do not leave unattended and seek medical help.

### Prolapsed eye ball

Meaning the eye is now in front of the lids and the optic nerve cord is being stretched as the lids swell. Never touch the eye ball. Treatment is as follows:

- Keep the eye moist at all costs. Use tap water soaked into a pad, squeeze out and apply to the eye area.
- Once moistened, soak the pad again in tap water and place gently over the eye.
- Hold or bandage in position.
- Do not leave unattended and stop any self-mutilation.
- Keep warm, quiet and comfort able.
- Seek veterinary assistance urgently.

The important point to remember is that the eye must not be allowed to dry out. Some breeds of dog are prone to eye prolapse due to their shortened faces, such as Pugs, Pekinese and Boxers. Therefore always use extra care when handling these breeds.

If the handler is present when the prolapse happens, return the eye by holding the upper and lower eye lids and pulling them gently over the eye ball. This is only possible immediately postinjury and do not attempt if the eye has been prolapsed for longer than ten minutes.

### Perforating injury

Seen when usually a sharp instrument becomes embedded in the structure of the eye. Never pull the foreign body out of the eye even if it is large enough to grasp. If it is removed non-surgically the front chamber of the eye would leak fluid (*aqueous humour*), causing the back chamber to prolapse forward, thereby destroying the eye structure.

Treatment is to keep the eye moist, prevent self-mutilation and get to the veterinary surgery quickly.

# Chapter 19
# Basic Bandaging

## Reasons for bandaging

- Protect a wound.
- Prevent self-mutilation and interference.
- Support soft tissues (muscle or ligament) in sprains and strains.
- Stop bleeding (pressure bandage).
- Prevent contamination.
- Reduce swelling (cold bandage or pack).
- Hold a dressing in place.

## Layers of a bandage

### Primary or contact layer

Dressings are placed against the wound to assist healing.

- *Adherent* dressings, i.e. gauze swab, tend to stick to the wound and may be difficult to remove without damaging a layer of new tissue.
- *Non-adherent* dressings, i.e. Melolin or Rondo, absorb wound fluids into cotton wool type backing. They do not stick to wounds or cause so much damage on removal.
- *Moist* dressings, i.e. Intrasite, encourage healing.

### Secondary layer

This provides the absorption and padding, i.e. cotton wool (Fig. 19.1).

### Top layer

Secures the above and protects them from the environment and the patient. This is either an adhesive or self-adherent material, i.e. Elastoplast or Vetrap (Fig. 19.2).

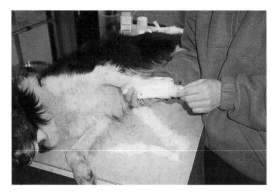

**Fig. 19.1**   The area to be bandaged is protected with a padding material, between the toes and dew claw.

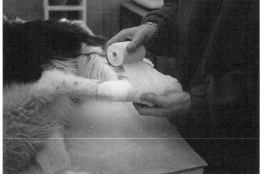

**Fig. 19.2**   A protective layer covers the bandage.

## Aims of bandaging

- It must be comfortable. If applied too tightly, the animal will try to remove the bandage or the surface tissues will be damaged by the animal's constant licking.
- Prevents the animal interfering with the area under the bandage.
- Limits movement in the case of broken bones or tissue damage and therefore limits pain.
- Stays on for the required amount of time.
- Looks neat but will do the job until professional help is reached.

---

**Watch out for:**

- Smells coming from the bandage
- Discomfort
- Interference or self-mutilation to try and remove the bandage
- Overexercising
- Bandage getting wet or dirty
- Any signs of ill health

If any of the above are seen in an animal with a bandage, report to the veterinary surgeon straight away for advice.

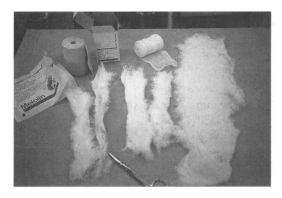

**Fig. 19.3**  Prepare all materials prior to restraint of the animal.

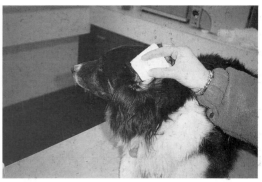

**Fig. 19.4**  Ear bandage. First protect the wound with a dressing.

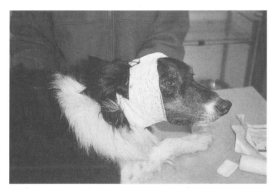

**Fig. 19.5**  Hold dressing in place with injured ear flap bandaged against the top of the head.

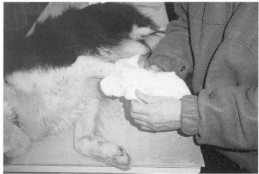

**Fig. 19.6**  The padding.

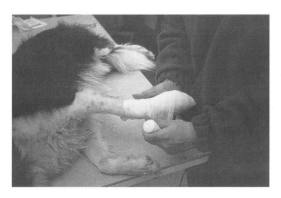

**Fig. 19.7**  The bandage.

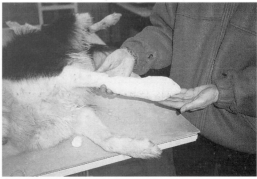

**Fig. 19.8**  The top protective layer.

# Rules for bandaging

- Wash hands before starting to prevent introducing infection.
- Get all the materials together before restraining the animal.
- Never stick adhesive tapes onto the animal's coat or hair as it is hard to remove.
- Do not use safety pins or elastic bands to secure the ends of any bandage. Use narrow adhesive tape on the bandage surface.
- In the case of a leg bandage, include the foot otherwise it will swell.
- Have the animal restrained in the correct position for application of the bandage.
- If unsure of temperament, always muzzle for safety.

Figs 19.3–19.8 demonstrate bandaging technique.

## *Application*

It is important to apply the bandage material in a spiral fashion to prevent development of pressure rings on the skin. A *pressure ring* happens when a bandage is applied in a circular manner or the bandage has slipped from its original position on the limb to lie as rings over one area.

A tight bandage can cause fluid to build up in the tissues and prevent its proper flow. To make sure a bandage is not applied too tightly, it should be possible to easily slip two fingers under the edge of the bandage.

# Chapter 20
# The Hospital Environment

Animals are hospitalised for:

- Observation
- Operation
- Treatment
- Collection of samples or to run diagnostic tests
- Nursing care

To ensure a high standard of care, there must be adequate facilities, equipment and trained human resources.

Locations within the practice for the care of patients include:

- Preparation room
- Preparation/triage room
- Kennels
- Intensive care areas
- Theatre
- Recovery area

## Environmental temperature

Most mammals and birds are able to regulate their body temperature to maintain optimum levels. The ideal temperature range varies between species to allow for the working of the internal environment of each, known as *homoeostasis*.

The monitoring of body temperature of cold-blooded species like snakes, lizards and other reptiles is not useful, because they are dependent on the environmental temperature for body function.

However, in the case of warm-blooded patients who control their own body temperature, help is sometimes needed. When conscious and healthy, control is generally good but when ill or injured, patients may need help from the nursing environment.

### Conditions causing a raised body temperature

- Heat stroke
- Infection
- Stress
- Exercise
- Poisons

### Conditions causing a lowered body temperature

- Very young/old
- Serious haemorrhage
- Shock
- Recovery from anaesthesia
- Poisons

Patients in the veterinary hospital will benefit, often dramatically, if the environmental temperature is raised or lowered to suit their special needs when, for a variety of reasons, they are unable to maintain it within normal limits themselves.

Methods to assist these patients include:

- Heat pads
- Bubble wrap
- Water-circulating pads
- Incubator
- Hot water bottles – well wrapped
- Lightweight blankets
- Space blankets
- Vet beds
- Bean bags

Whatever the normal body temperature – maintain it!

## Hygiene and cleaning

The hospital environment will house high concentrations of micro-organisms which are potentially *pathogenic* (can cause disease) to patients. Injured or diseased patients are at risk because of decreased resistance to infection. Every effort must be made to decrease the microbe population in the hospital environment in order to safeguard patients.

In order to protect the patient:

- Eliminate or control source of the disease – disinfectant and antiseptic use.
- Increase host resistance to disease – vaccination, improve diet.
- Prevent transmission of disease – ventilation, isolation of suspect animals, use of disposable protective clothing.

If mops are used for washing the floor (Fig. 20.1), the rules below should be followed:

- Mop heads should be washed in the washing machine and dried daily.
- If used more than once daily, soak for 30 minutes in a bucket of disinfectant.
- Never leave in soaking solution for more than 30 minutes.
- Wring out thoroughly before use on the floors.

In use, the mop should be moved from left to right across the body, never pushed back and forward in front of the operator. Agitate in the disinfectant solution, wring out and proceed to clean. When the area around the operator has been cleaned, then move, repeating the mop rinsing. Start with the area farthest from the door and do not allow anyone to walk on the floor until it is dry.

Change the disinfectant solution between rooms or more frequently if heavily soiled. Use a separate mop and cleaning equipment in the sterile areas such as the theatre suite.

---

**Routine room cleaning**

- Remove waste from all bins and replace plastic liner.
- Clean and disinfect walls.
- Spot clean surfaces, cupboard doors, doors, light fixtures, drip stands and any other items routinely kept in this area.
- Check and restock any disposable equipment.
- Clean and disinfect the sinks.
- Clean and disinfect the floor.
- Disinfect and store cleaning equipment.

---

Different hospital areas require different approaches. The following areas are important:

- Consultation rooms
- Kennels/recovery area
- Triage
- Theatre

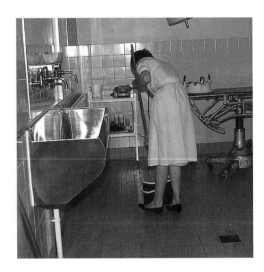

**Fig. 20.1**   Cleaning the floor area in the theatre.

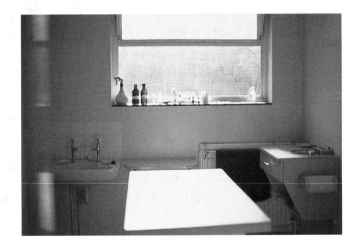

**Fig. 20.2**   Consultation room.

## Consultation rooms (Fig. 20.2)

- Clean and disinfect all floors and surfaces at the end of the consultation periods (morning, afternoon and evening).
- Collect used instruments, wash and leave ready for sterilising (if appropriate).
- Dispose of all waste, using the correct disposal bags (yellow for clinical waste).
- Use disposable cloth or paper towel only.
- Disinfect all surfaces.
- Empty bins.

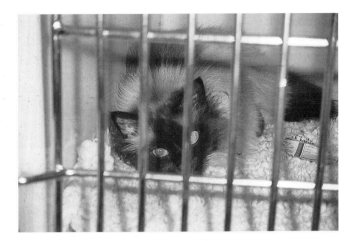

**Fig. 20.3**   Recovery cage.

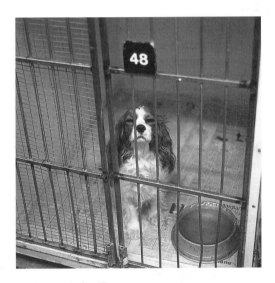

**Fig. 20.4**   Numbering of kennels for ID purposes.

## *Kennels/recovery area (Fig. 20.3)*

This area includes the room maintenance and the cage/kennel maintenance. Room maintenance is as for routine cleaning instructions, to be carried out at a time which would cause the least disturbance to inpatients as possible. This may be early in the morning before surgery begins or overnight if the hospital has night shift staff.

If an animal is recovering from procedures, disturb as little as possible but if soiled, clean out and make comfortable straight away.

Check before disposal of waste materials that a sample is not required (the cage/kennel should be numbered or carry a cage/kennel card) (Fig. 20.4). If a

# Chapter 21
# The Hospitalised Patient

## Records and monitoring

Records contain owner/pet details and other information which is vital to the veterinary surgeon who must assess the patient's progress (Fig. 21.1).

- Temperature, pulse and respiration rates taken as often as necessary
- Detail on appetite and feeding
- Urine/faeces passed
- Any vomiting episodes

## Observation

The veterinary surgeon will examine at least twice daily to assess progress. The nursing staff are then responsible for the animal's cleanliness, feeding, watering, medication at correct times and reports on any changes to its condition. The contact time due to the above duties allows nursing staff to:

- Observe the patient
- Notice any behavioural changes
- Note quantity of food eaten and which is its favourite food
- Give detail on whether the faeces is formed or diarrhoeal
- Note if the animal coughs after waking up
- Note whether the animal shows signs of pain or discomfort

## Feeding and watering

The cage or kennel should contain a support for feed and water bowls, to prevent them being tipped over. Bowls are always washed and disinfected daily. Fresh water is always available unless prohibited by the veterinary surgeon in charge of the case. A sign is then placed on the front of the housing indicating the patient should not be fed (Fig. 21.2).

Special patients may require measured amounts of water, so that water input and output can be recorded (Fig. 21.3).

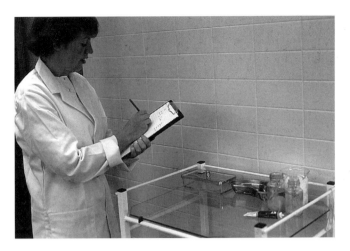

**Fig. 21.1**   Recording information on patients.

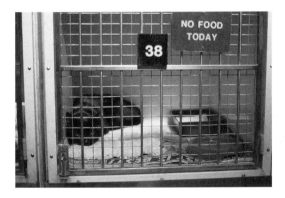

**Fig. 21.2**   Identify kennels where restrictions are instructed by the attending veterinary surgeon.

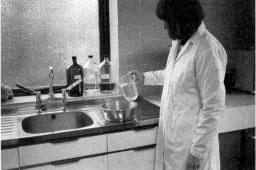

**Fig. 21.3**   Measure the required amount and record on the record chart.

Feeding varies with patients but is normally twice daily, as per the hospital routine:

- In the morning to determine the appetite
- In order to assist in the administration of some medicines
- In the case of medical diabetes mellitus, where medicines and food must be timed and regulated
- Postoperatively, patients may need to be encouraged to feed (Fig. 21.4)

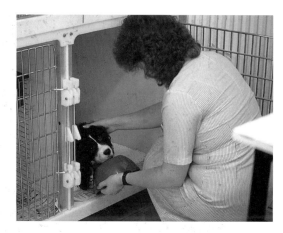

**Fig. 21.4**  Postoperatively patients will need to be encouraged to feed.

Feeding may also be contraindicated for a number of reasons:

- Scheduled for surgery and must have an empty stomach
- Medical condition
- After surgery to the gastrointestinal tract
- Requires blood tests
- Is vomiting and/or has diarrhoea

## Hygiene

Regular checks are made through the day to make sure no animal lies in a body discharge (Fig. 21.5). After moving the animal from a soiled housing or kennel, check to see if samples need to be collected for investigations.

Mark the cage details, with collection times, then clean and disinfect. To prevent animals from getting soiled, grills may be covered with a layer of bedding to allow a soak-away effect for use with incontinence pads.

## Temperature control

Pre- and postoperative patients need assistance to regain lost body heat and prevent the establishing of shock. Heat can be provided by:

- Environmental thermostat controls
- Kennels with underfloor heating
- Heated underpads (Fig. 21.6)
- Incubator for small or newborn animals

It is important never to overheat but simply to support body temperature. Use of heat lamps can be harmful if the animal is unable to move away; it could

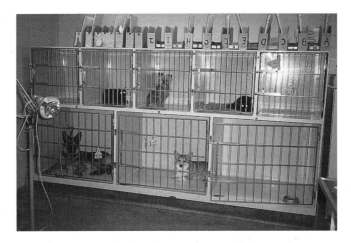

**Fig. 21.5**   Hospital holding kennels allow easy monitoring for signs of soiling.

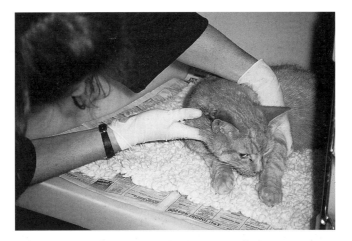

**Fig. 21.6**   Bedding for warmth postoperatively will support body temperature.

overheat and even suffer skin burns if the lamp is too close. Always keep the lamp a minimum of one metre from the body of the animal to avoid any overheating or burns.

## Recumbent patients

- Use deep bedding to prevent pressure on any bony areas (Fig. 21.7)
- Do not allow to remain in soiled kennel
- Use incontinence pads
- Assist drinking to prevent dehydration
- Assist eating, giving small meals often
- Groom and clean away any food on the coat after feeding

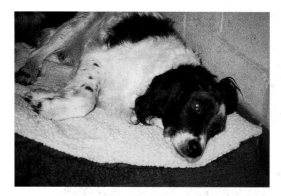

**Fig. 21.7** Plenty of bedding for recumbent patients.

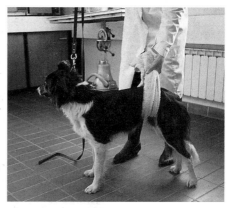

**Fig. 21.8** Assist to stand using sling to support hindquarters.

- Unless contraindicated, encourage limb movements to stimulate circulation (Fig. 21.8)
- Turn the animal every 1–2 hours to prevent fluid pooling in the chest due to shallow breathing
- Rub and stroke body to stimulate surface circulation, generating heat and fluid movement within the tissues
- Spend time playing with the animal
- Assist to urinate or check indwelling urinary catheter

## Handling

Use coat care and grooming as an excuse to handle. Also wipe any discharges from nose, eye or ears and keep the area around the mouth moistened using damp cotton wool to simulate the animal's own grooming routines. This will all contribute to a feeling of well-being for the animal, accustoms them to the nursing staff and promotes recovery.

## Isolation and barrier nursing

If the patient has a suspected contagious or zoonotic disease, it must be moved to the isolation area. Barrier nursing follows strict rules to prevent crossinfection between routine patients or staff members. Barrier nursing involves:

- Protective clothing – disposable apron, intact gloves and mask if necessary
- Change of footwear
- Required drugs and medical equipment for patient care

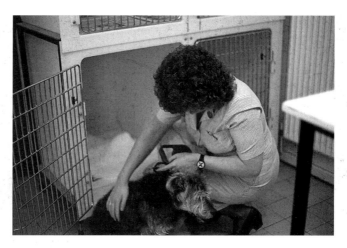

**Fig. 21.9**   TLC to promote recovery.

- Cleaning equipment for unit use only
- Feeding materials and cleaning of bowls in the unit
- One member of staff to work in isolation only and not handle any other patients

## Medication

For any patient in the hospital, always check:

- Timings
- Dosage per day
- Whether tablet or injection required and/or assistance
- Route

## Fluid therapy

This will involve:

- Care and maintenance of intravenous catheters
- Preventing patient interference (use of Elizabethan collar)
- Checking the fluid is running in properly
- Monitoring quantities delivered
- Changing drip fluid bags on instruction
- Monitoring hydration status
- Recording and reporting all details

## Environmental enrichment

- Preferred foods
- Assisting to eat and drink; expect this to be time consuming but time well spent
- Comfort in the cage, kennel or housing
- Enough space
- Music helps calm both humans and animals
- Do not mix species
- Toys are helpful for long-stay patients, providing interest and, if not contraindicated, activity too
- TLC (Fig. 21.9)

# Chapter 22
# Monitoring Temperature, Pulse and Respiration

The skill of observation and monitoring life signs is essential to nursing of any species of animal. It involves the comparing of normal behaviour against that which is abnormal. Time spent with an animal, using all senses, is most important. The nurse should be capable of recognising minute changes to the animal's life signs and temperament.

Temperature, pulse and respiration or breathing all vary in animals due to environmental temperature, recent exercise, stress situations and excitement. Increase or decrease in the rate of these life signs can also indicate a problem with a body system or that a disease is present. These life signs should be checked hourly or, until an animal is stabilised, more frequently.

## Temperature

Most species can regulate their body temperature in response to internal and external influences to within a very narrow range, due to homoeostasis. Taking the body temperature of cold-blooded species like reptiles is not useful because they rely on environmental sources for their own heat. The ability of warm-blooded animals to control their own body temperature may disappear when ill or injured.

### Heat loss methods

- Sweating
- Panting
- Drinking water
- Position – spread out, seeking a cold surface to lie on
- Vasodilation – surface blood vessels increase in size to lose body heat

### Heat gain methods

- Shivering
- Position – curled up
- Vasoconstriction – surface blood vessels reduce in size to reduce body heat loss

Temperature is assessed by:

- Touching extremities
- Body position
- Thermometer reading

## Rules

- Take the temperature at the very least twice a day (it is always lower after sleep).
- Leave the thermometer in position for at least one minute; in the case of the subclinical thermometer, leave in position for at least two minutes.
- After insertion into the rectum, tilt the thermometer to contact the epithelial wall lining the tract. This ensures that the thermometer is not placed into faeces in the rectum, which would give a false reading.

## Taking the temperature

---

**Equipment required to take a temperature**

- Thermometer
- Lubricant such as KY Jelly or medicinal liquid paraffin
- Small amount of cotton wool
- Antiseptic water-based solution
- Watch with a second hand

---

(1) Collect and prepare all required equipment.
(2) Correctly restrain patient (second person restraining head).
(3) Shake down the thermometer and check the reading.
(4) Apply the lubricant to the thermometer.
(5) Insert into the rectum for the correct length of time (never be tempted to reduce this time).
(6) Remove, wipe with the cotton wool and read.
(7) Wipe clean using antiseptic solution.

Store the thermometer in a jar or container containing dilute water-based antiseptic solution.

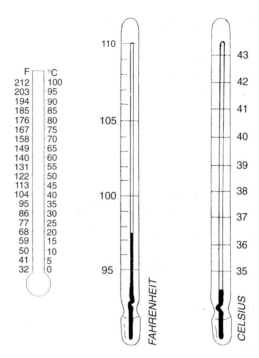

**Fig. 22.1** Thermometer scales.

- Always wipe clean of faecal material before placing in the jar or container.
- Protect the bulb end of the thermometer by placing a layer of cotton wool at the bottom of the container.
- Never store or clean in a hot solution as this could damage the thermometer.
- Before use, wipe clean of the antiseptic solution which could irritate the rectal lining.

Always write down the reading so that a record can be built up of any changes that occurred, at what stage of the disease and the time of day.

Types of thermometer in use include:

- Celsius or centigrade – with a scale reading of 35–43 (Fig. 22.1)
- Fahrenheit – with a scale reading of 94–108 (Fig. 22.1)
- Subclinical Celsius – with a scale reading of 25–40

The formula for converting Celsius to Fahrenheit is as follows.

F to C – Subtract 32, multiply by 5, divide by 9.
C to F – multiply by 9, divide by 5, add 32.

Normal temperatures.

| Species | Celsius | Fahrenheit |
|---------|---------|------------|
| Dog | 38.3–38.7 | 100.9–101.7 |
| Cat | 38.0–38.5 | 100.4–101.6 |
| Guinea pig | 38.4–40 | 102.2–104 |
| Rabbit | 38.5–40 | 101.5–104 |
| Rat | 37.5 | 99.9 |
| Hamster | 36–38 | 98–101 |
| Mouse | 37.5 | 99.5 |

Differences between:

**Clinical thermometer**

Contains mercury
Triangular in shape
Scale difference
Constriction near bulb
Needs to be shaken down before use
Short shaft

**Laboratory thermometer**

Contains spirit or mercury
Circular in shape
Scale difference
No constriction
Needs no shaking down before use
Long shaft

Temperature increase may be seen:

- In infections and fevers
- After recent exercise
- In fear or excitement
- In heat stroke (*hyperthermia*)
- In hot weather

Temperature decrease may be seen:

- In shock and severe bleeding
- In exposure cases (*hypothermia*)
- In hibernation
- In anaesthesia
- Before impending death (moribund animal)
- Immediately before *parturition* (giving birth)

## Pulse

The pulse is used as a means of checking the heart (*cardio*) and blood (*vascular*) function. With each heart beat, the artery walls expand and contract in size to allow the created wave of blood to pass and maintain its speed of flow. This is called the pulse. If there is a change in the heart function or the volume of blood then there will be a reflected change in the pulse rate (speed) or character.

Words used to describe the pulse include:

- Intermittent
- Thready – slow, soft pulse
- Irregular
- Strong
- Weak

A normal pulse is usually described as regular, strong or firm. It is essential that time is spent feeling pulses, both normal and abnormal, to increase the operator's ability to assess the state of the animal. This will also dramatically decrease the time it takes to find the animal's pulse.

The pulse is taken where an artery runs close to the body surface. Each pulsation corresponds with the contraction of the right and left ventricles of the heart.

### Sites used

- Femoral artery located in the groin region on the medial aspect of the femur of the hind leg.
- Digital artery located on the cranial or anterior surface of the hock region of the hind leg.
- Coccygeal artery located on the ventral (underside) aspect of the base of the tail just above the rectum.
- Lingual artery located on the ventral (underside) aspect of the tongue. However, this site can only be used in unconscious or anaesthetised animals.

The most common site used to take the pulse is the femoral artery on the hind leg. Before taking the pulse, the animal must be suitably restrained so two people make the task much easier.

### Taking the pulse

- Get the animal used to being restrained.
- Once the animal is settled, take the pulse by placing the fingers over the chosen artery.
- When properly located, using a watch with a second hand, count the pulse for one minute. Never shorten this period because the pulse can change quickly and a reading of less than one minute could be inaccurate and therefore useless.
- Write down the pulse count at the end of the minute.
- Relax the restraint of the animal and praise.

Normal pulse recording.

| Species | Pulse rate (beats per minute) |
| --- | --- |
| Dog | 60–180* |
| Cat | 110–180 |
| Rabbit | 150–300 |
| Guinea pig | 230–320 |
| Hamster | 300–600 |
| Mouse | 500–600 |

*The pulse range in dogs is due to the size variation from toy breeds (nearer the 180 end of the range) to giant breeds (nearer the 60 end of the range).

**Pulse terms**

*Dysrhythmia* – indicates that the pulse and heart rate are not synchronised. The pulse is lower due to the heart pumping blood inefficiently.
*Sinus arrhythmia* – refers to the pulse rate increase on breathing in and decrease on breathing out. This is often considered to be normal.
*Fast pulse* – occurs when the tissues are not getting enough oxygen and the heart is compensating by speeding up to meet the body's needs. Fast pulse can be normal after exercise.

**Pulse increase**

- Exercise
- Excitement or stress
- Heart/valve disease
- Shock or loss of blood
- Pain
- High temperature/fever

**Pulse decrease**

- Sleep
- Unconsciousness
- Heart disease
- Other disease condition

Normal respiration rates.

| Species | Rate (breaths per minute) |
| --- | --- |
| Dog | 10–30 |
| Cat | 20–30 |
| Rabbit | 35–65 |
| Guinea pig | 110–150 |
| Hamster | 75 |
| Gerbil | 90–140 |
| Mouse | 100–250 |

# Respiration

Normal breathing is almost silent, although air flow may be heard in the airways. The breathing and cardiovascular systems are very closely linked so a change in one is mirrored in the other. If the blood gas levels of oxygen or carbon dioxide become abnormal this will be seen in the animal's colour, its pulse rate and character and in the breathing.

Certain breeds of dog and cat may, because of airway anatomy (short-nosed breeds), make considerable breathing sounds and this is normal.

There should be a rhythm to the breathing, in that the time between breathing in and out should be equal. The breathing can be varied by use of the voluntary or skeletal muscles of the chest or thorax.

The ability to voluntarily alter breathing means that the rate can only be taken once the animal has settled. Any obvious restraint will probably cause the breathing to increase in response. The reading is taken on either breathing in or breathing out and when the animal:

- Is not panting
- Has not recently exercised
- Has not been stressed by overrestraint
- Is not asleep

The respiratory rate is taken when the animal is calm, awake and comfortable. After close observation by the operator, a decision is taken to count on breathing in or breathing out. The recording is timed using a watch with a second hand for one minute. Note is also made of the depth of breathing.

*Causes of respiration increase*

- Shock or haemorrhage
- Recent exercise
- Pain
- Excitement or fear

- Heat stroke
- Medical disease, especially of the respiratory system

*Causes of respiration decrease*

- Unconsciousness
- Sleep
- Poisons
- Low body temperature (hypothermia)

---

**Breathing terms**

- *Tachypnoea* – rapid, shallow breathing.
- *Hyperpnoea* – panting.
- *Apnoea* – no breathing taking place.
- *Cheyne–Stokes* – irregular breathing (deep breaths, then fast shallow breaths) seen shortly before death.
- *Dyspnoea* – difficulty breathing in or out and often painful.

---

*Signs of difficult breathing*

- Forced breathing out
- Flaring of nostrils
- Extended head and neck
- Elbows rotated away from the chest
- Breathing through the mouth
- Exaggerated movements of the chest and abdomen
- Sounds
- Unable to settle

# Chapter 23
# Pharmacy and the Administration of Drugs

Pharmacology is the science of drugs:

- The way in which the drug affects the body
- Its absorption into the body
- Its metabolism by the body
- The method used by the body to finally excrete it

Dispensing is the giving out of drugs to the owner of the animal requiring them, either by the veterinary practice at which the owner is registered or by taking a prescription to a dispensing chemist.

Drugs are administered in various ways. This is often dependent on the drug target in the body, how quickly the effect of the drug is required and the ability of the owner to give the drug.

## Routes

### Oral (Fig. 23.1)

This is the most frequently used route for drugs because the owner can treat at home. The products are supplied in various forms, from tablet to powder. Many tablets have an outer coating and therefore should never be broken up or crushed in case the action of the drug is reduced. Reasons for coating tablets include:

- Protection of the drug from moisture
- To hide an unpleasant taste
- To assist in identification
- To protect the drug from the hydrochloric acid in the stomach (enteric coated)
- Protection of the stomach from the irritant effect of a drug

Oral administration can have disadvantages.

- If the animal is vomiting
- Absorption can be slow and some of the drug may not be absorbed at all
- The presence of food may reduce the drug's effect
- The animal may refuse to swallow the drug
- Owner is unable to give the drug to the animal

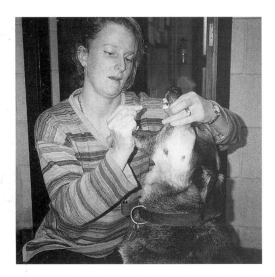

**Fig. 23.1** The mouth is opened wide so that the tablet can then be placed at the back of the throat for swallowing.

### Parenteral

A route other than by mouth. It usually refers to or is taken to mean 'by injection'. Any drug administered by this method must be sterile and the method involves some skin site cleaning and personal hygiene. The most frequently used injection methods are:

- *Subcutaneous* – into the connective tissues below the skin (below the hypodermis). This method is for non-irritant drugs and absorption is slow.
- *Intramuscular* – directly into a muscle body (hind leg or back). This method is used for small volumes of drug only and can be painful but the drug is more rapidly absorbed than by the subcutaneous route.
- *Intravenous* – into a surface vein (foreleg, hind leg or neck vein). This method places the drug directly into the bloodstream and has very rapid action.

Other injection routes less frequently used are:

- *Epidural* – into the vertebral canal to give spinal pain control (*analgesia*)
- *Intra-articular* – directly into a joint
- *Intradermal* – into the skin structure

### Topical

These drug preparations are applied to a surface tissue like the skin, eyes or ears (Fig. 23.2). They are absorbed into either just the surface of the skin or mucous membranes or the structure of the skin, depending on the material used to carry the drug. Some topical drugs may be able to move into body systems which is

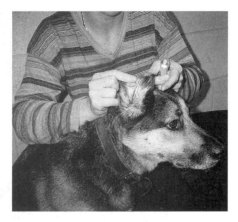

**Fig. 23.2**  The ointment/cream is applied to the affected area on the ear flap.

why the operator must immediately wash off any drug that contacts their skin. Types of carriers used include:

- Water to place wettable powder against the skin
- Petroleum jelly as ointment that melts with body heat
- Oil and water together as a cream, which will penetrate into the skin layers
- Detergent-based products as medicated shampoos to cover the skin surface before rinsing off

## Pharmacology and dispensing

For safe drug administration, be sure that the following are checked and confirmed before medication is given.

---

**Is it the right:**

- drug?
- patient?
- dose?
- route for the drug?
- time interval?

---

### Administer the right drug

- Check label
- Check against the animal's medical record, if available
- If the writing is illegible on the medical record, get it clarified
- Understand the difference between trade names and generic names

### Administer the right drug to the right patient

- Check the ID on the animal
- Check the ID on the kennel
- Check any medical records

### Administer the right dose

- Read instructions
- Check with supervising member of staff

### Administer the drug by the correct route

- Know the meaning of abbreviations like:
  i.m. – intramuscular
  p.o. – by mouth (per os)
  i.v. – intravenous
  s.c. – subcutaneous
- Do not crush 'delayed action' capsules/tablets to mix with food
- Some drugs must be given i.m. for absorption as they may be irritant given s.c., so always check the instructions on the container or product leaflet

### Administer the drug at the right time

- Know the abbreviations:
  b.i.d. or b.d. – twice daily or every 12 hours
  t.i.d. or t.d. – three times daily or every eight hours
  q.i.d. or q.d. – four times daily or every six hours
- Observe the drug intervals for best therapeutic levels

### Document drug administration on the animal's records

- The drug, dose, route, site of administration, date and time
- If there is no recording, assume the drug has not been given
- Record after drug is given, not before, in case of problems

### Be aware of drug / food or drug / drug interactions

- Some drugs must be given with food, like aspirin
- Some drugs must be given on an empty stomach, like the antibiotic ampicillin
- Drug interactions when treating for heart disease, arthritis and epilepsy
- Record any adverse effects seen

# Labels for drug containers

For legal requirements the essential information on a container label is:

- Veterinary practice name and address
- Date of dispensing
- Owner's name and address
- The words KEEP OUT OF REACH OF CHILDREN
- The words FOR ANIMAL TREATMENT ONLY
- If applicable, the words FOR EXTERNAL USE ONLY

Additional useful information that may be included is:

- Drug strength, for example 50 mg amoxycillin
- Trade name (licensed name for use only by the manufacturing company that developed the drug) or *generic* name (drug chemical name and manufactured by various drug companies)
- Animal's name
- Directions for use; for example, 'give twice daily'

---

Warnings should also be attached to certain drugs such as aspirin in full-strength form (150 mg). Labels should read 'Unsuitable for cats'. This drug can be used in humans and dogs but in cats its effect lasts a lot longer. If a second dose is given by the owner too soon then the cat will be overdosed. Clearance time for aspirin is:

- Humans – four hours
- Dogs – eight hours
- Cats – 30 hours

---

# Handling and dispensing drugs

## Legal aspects

Drugs used in the treatment of animals are classified under the Medicines Act of 1968 into four groups:

(1) POM – these are prescription-only medicines; only doctors, dentists and veterinary surgeons can prescribe them and dispensing is either via the veterinary surgeon or a pharmacist.

(2) PML – these are called pharmacy and merchants list medicines. They are licensed products for use only in animals and can be supplied by veterinary

practices, saddlers and animal wholesale outlets such as animal feed and farm merchants.

(3)   P – these are pharmacy medicines supplied by veterinary practices and dispensing chemist chains.

(4)   GSL – these are general sales list medicines and can be supplied and sold by pet shops and other outlets.

The group symbol is found on the drug container label and any outer packaging.

A special category of drugs, those that could be abused by humans, are known as the *controlled drugs* (CD). The legislation applicable here is the Misuse of Drugs Regulations 1985, which is divided into five schedules. These schedules are set out in decreasing order of the need to control.

* *Schedule 1* – includes drugs like cannabis and hallucinogenic drugs such as LSD, which are considered non-therapeutic and are therefore not legally held in veterinary practice for the purpose of treating animals.
* *Schedule 2* – includes the opiate analgesics (pain control) like morphine pethidine, and etorphine (anaesthetic agent). These drugs are POM and records are kept on their ordering, supply, safe storage and, if out of date or not required, their destruction.
* *Schedule 3* – includes barbiturates (used for anaesthesia, control of epilepsy and euthanasia), some minor stimulant drugs and some analgesics (pain control). These drugs are POM and must have safe storage and purchase records.
* *Schedule 4* – includes the benzodiazepine drugs such as valium and diazepam (used to reduce stress). When these drugs are given to patients within the veterinary practice (for example, in injectable form only) they are exempt from restrictions.
* *Schedule 5* – contains preparations with only traces of otherwise controlled drugs, such as cocaine, codeine (cough mixture) and morphine (kaolin and morphine for diarrhoea treatment). The levels of drug are so small that they are exempt from restrictions.

Some drugs carry special risks. Harmful products may produce an acute effect immediately after contact whereas others may accumulate over time and constant exposure will be necessary before their effect on the operator or nurse is seen.

High-risk products include:

* Certain hormone products, like those used to postpone oestrus
* Cytotoxic drugs – those used in the treatment of cancers
* Gaseous anaesthetic agents like halothane
* Certain antibiotics
* Antifungal powders – those used to treat ringworm
* Insecticides

# Drugs glossary

| Group | Definition |
|---|---|
| Anabolic | Promotes growth of body tissue |
| Analgesic | Relieves or prevents pain |
| Anthelmintic | Kills internal parasitic worms |
| Antibiotic | Disrupts or destroys bacteria |
| Anticoagulant | Prevents blood from clotting |
| Antidiuretic | Hormone which reduces urine output |
| Corticosteroids | Suppress inflammation |
| Diuretic | Increases urine production |
| Emetic | Causes vomiting |
| Sedative | Reduces awareness of surroundings |
| Vaccine | Stimulates the production of antibodies |

# Chapter 24
# Isolation and Quarantine

## Isolation

Isolation is required when an animal is believed to have or has a disease which can be passed on to others (*contagious*). There is also protective isolation for susceptible animals, e.g. unvaccinated puppies and kittens. In their case, the isolation is in the owner's home and garden, which becomes the controlled environment.

In many veterinary practices and hospitals there is a purpose-built isolation unit where contagious animals can be housed and nursed. In other types of group housing, this type of facility may have to be created, as the need arises. Home-made isolation may involve use of a foldaway cage or cage box in a non-animal area of the unit which can be carefully controlled.

---

**Infectious diseases of the dog and cat needing isolation**

| Dog | Cat |
|---|---|
| Distemper | Feline infectious peritonitis |
| Hepatitis | Feline leukaemia virus |
| Leptospirosis | Feline panleucopenia |
| Kennel cough | Cat flu |
| Ringworm | Ringworm |
| Sarcoptic mange | |

---

The affected animal is housed in such a manner as to prevent other animals coming into contact with the disease-producing organisms it will be shedding. Micro-organisms can be shed via:

- Urine
- Faeces
- Blood
- Discharges from eyes, ears, nose, mouth, prepuce, vulva or a wound

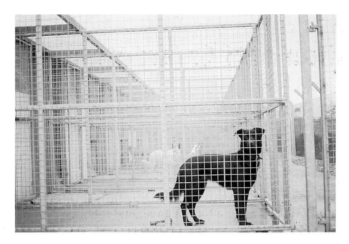

**Fig. 24.1**  The dog is kept isolated from others in its own housing and run area.

- Respiratory tract via sneezing or coughing
- Vomit

Bearing in mind the exit routes for contagious diseases, isolation must follow disease management rules:

- One member of staff specifically allocated to the isolation area
- Change into protective clothing
- Change into protective footwear or set up a footbath containing disinfectant
- The unit must contain all required food preparation equipment and food bowls
- Cleaning equipment used only in the unit
- Additional protection of gloves and mask
- Instruments used here are cleaned here
- Safe disposal of soiled bedding, faeces, urine, etc.
- Medical supplies available

All staff members must disinfect or change footwear, change overall and wash hands in antiseptic solution before leaving to move through the other areas of the animal housing. It is essential never to put healthy animals or humans at risk by careless behaviour. There is also the possibility that the disease may transmit from animals to human carers (known as a *zoonone* or *zoonotic disease*).

## Quarantine

This refers to the detention of animals for a set period of time, in isolation from other animals, in order to screen for disease (Fig. 24.1).

In the UK, quarantine refers to the detention of animals coming into the country and the time will vary depending on the species involved. For dogs and cats, the time is six calendar months to be spent in a quarantine kennel in order to screen for rabies in particular. For other species, the times and locations vary but will involve separation from the main group of animals or birds at a given location. In this manner, the resident animals are not put at risk by the newcomer.

### New proposals for the quarantine of dogs and cats in the UK

In March 1999 the government's proposed changes to the quarantine laws, as recommended by the Kennedy Advisory Group, were published. The Kennedy Advisory Group was appointed to look at the existing regulations and make recommendations for replacing quarantine. The government intends to introduce the Kennedy-style arrangements by April 2001.

The new scheme proposes to allow dogs and cats coming from EU countries, certain other European countries and rabies-free islands to enter the UK without having to undergo quarantine, provided they can meet the necessary criteria regarding vaccination and identification.

These changes would not apply to dogs and cats entering the UK from the USA or Canada.

Requirements for entry under the new rules are as follows:

* Must be permanently identified with electronic microchip.
* Vaccinated against rabies using an inactivated vaccine.
* Treated for exotic diseases not in the UK, i.e. parasitic infections.
* Have an official health certificate containing details of:
  – owner or keeper
  – identification and description of animal
  – vaccination record and booster information
  – blood tests and results
  – treatment for parasitic infections.

These regulations will be enforced by:

* Pre-entry checks by train operators, ferry companies and airlines.
* Random spot checks on animals arriving in the UK by the MAFF and official carriers.

# Appendix
# Anatomy and Physiology Terminology

The majority of terms referring to the body systems and medical conditions are derived from Greek or Latin. Most of these terms are a combination of two or more word parts. When they combine to become a word, they usually indicate some or all of the following:

- Body tissues involved
- What has gone wrong
- Quantity (a lot or very little)
- Levels of infection or inflammation
- Colour or substance
- Fluid involved

You may find it helpful to practise defining the components of the words separately, then combine them to find out the meaning of the complete word. In many ways it is no different from learning a new language and by memorising the common beginnings and endings, the rest can be worked out. It is always helpful to have a veterinary dictionary for the less frequently used terms and words.

## Medical terminology

Certain syllables are commonly used as the beginning or ending of medical terms, in many cases being added to a word stem which refers to a particular organ or part of the body.

- *Prefix* – beginning of a word stem
- *Suffix* – ending of a word stem

### Prefixes in anatomy/physiology

**A** or **An** – lack of, e.g. anaemia (lack of blood cells)
**Dys** – difficult or defective, e.g. dysphagia (difficulty swallowing)
**Endo** – within, e.g. endoscope (equipment used to look at working organs)
**Ex** – out, e.g. excision (to remove)

**Haema** or **Haemo** – refers to blood, e.g. haemorrhage (loss of blood)
**Hyper** – excess of, e.g. hyperthermia (high body temperature)
**Hypo** – lack of, e.g. hypothermia (low body temperature)
**Poly** – many or much, e.g. polydipsia (drinking a lot)
**Pyo** – pus, e.g. pyometra (pus-filled uterus)
**Sub** – beneath or under, e.g. sublingual (under the tongue)

*Suffixes in anatomy/physiology*

**itis** – inflammation, e.g. arthritis (inflammation of a joint)
**logy** – science or study of, e.g. dermatology (study of the skin)
**penia** – deficiency, e.g. leucopenia (deficiency of white blood cells)
**phagia** – eating, e.g. coprophagia (eating faeces)
**rrhoea** – increased discharge, e.g. diarrhoea (increased discharge of faeces)

## Word use

The following common words may help to illustrate the prefix/suffix idea:

- *Nephritis* – **neph** refers to the specialised cell of the kidney, known as the nephron; **itis** refers to inflammation of a tissue. The meaning of this word is kidney cell inflammation and pain.
- *Arthritis* – **arth** refers to a joint; **itis** means inflammation. The meaning of this word is joint inflammation and pain.
- *Hepatitis* – **hepat** refers to the specialised cell of the liver know as the hepatocyte; **itis** means inflammation. This word means inflammation and pain of the liver cells.
- *Haematoma* – **haem** refers to blood; **toma** refers to a lump or swelling. The meaning of this word is blood-filled lump or swelling.

These words are descriptions, not diagnoses, and simply refer to a tissue type or organ and what is happening to it.

## Anatomical directions

Anatomical directions are used to describe areas of the animal body. They are part of the language of medicine used between colleagues for communication. Many of these words originated from Greek or Latin.

The first four words are another way of saying above, below, front and back and are in common use when case recording in the medical world:

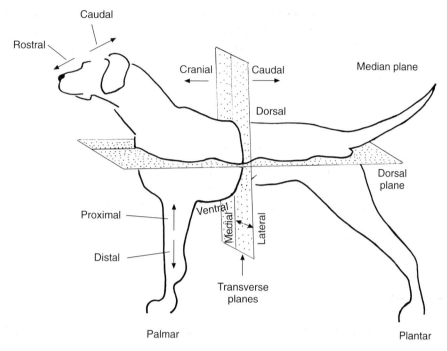

**Fig. A.1** Anatomical diections. Adapted from McBride, D.F. (1996) *Learning Veterinary Terminology*. Mosby, St Louis.

- *Dorsal* – towards the top or back surface of the body
- *Ventral* – towards the underside, lower surface or nearer the ground
- *Cranial or anterior* – situated at the front of the body or towards the head end
- *Caudal or posterior* – situated towards the back end of the body or towards the tail

Words to indicate side, middle or near the nose are:

- *Lateral* – to the side (left or right) or away from the middle of the body
- *Medial* – the midline of a body structure or the body
- *Rostral* – on the head but towards the nose

Words indicating near or far from a named body structure (especially limbs) are:

- *Proximal* – near to the body trunk or closer to a named structure
- *Distal* – away from the body trunk or further from a named structure

Words which describe where on a limb, surface, especially lower limb, surfaces are:

- *Palmar or volar* – indicating the caudal or back surface of the fore-limb, below the carpus or wrist area
- *Plantar* – indicating the caudal or back surface of the hind limb, below the tarsus or hock area

Words indicating inside or outside are:

- *Internal* – inside the body
- *External* – outside or surface

# Selected Reading

SECTION 1

**Animal Science**

Beckett, B.S. (1993) *Biology*. Oxford University Press, Oxford.

Blood, D.C. & Studdert, V.P. (1998) *Comprehensive Veterinary Dictionary*. Baillière Tindall, London.

Clegg, C. (1990) *Biology*. Heinemann, Oxford.

Jones, G. (1991) *Biology*. Cambridge University Press, Cambridge.

Lane, D. & Cooper, B. (1999) *Veterinary Nursing*. Pergamon Press, Oxford.

Michell, A.R. & Watkins, P.E. (1989) *Introduction to Veterinary Anatomy and Physiology*. BSAVA, Cheltenham.

Roberts, M.B.V. (1995) *Biology: A Functional Approach*. Nelson, London.

**Genetics**

Grossman, A. (1992) *The Standard Book of Dog Breeding*. Doral, Wilsonville, USA.

Nicholas, F.W. (1991) *Veterinary Genetics*. Oxford Science, Oxford.

Taylor, D. (1986) *You and Your Dog*. Dorling Kindersley, London.

Taylor, D. (1986) *You and Your Cat*. Dorling Kindersley, London.

SECTION 2

Ackerman, D.L. (n.d.) *Cat Health*. TFH, USA.

Alderton, D. (1986) *Rabbits and Guinea Pigs – Petkeeper Guide*. Salamander, London.

Alderton, D. (1989) *The Dog Care Manual*. Stanley Paul.

Anderson, R.S. & Edney, A.T.B. (1990) *Practical Animal Handling*. Pergamon Press, Oxford.

Barrie, A. (1987) *Step by Step – Guinea Pigs*. TFH, USA.

Bell, J.C., Palmer, S.R. & Payne, J.M. (1988) *The Zoonoses*. Edward Arnold, London.

Burger, I. (1993) *The Waltham Book of Companion Animal Nutrition*. Pergamon Press, Oxford.

Colville, J. (1991) *Diagnostic Parasitology for Veterinary Technicians*. American Veterinary Publications, California.

Evans, J.M. & White, K. (1994) *Book of the Bitch*. Henston, Guildford.

Evans, J.M. & White, K. (1994) *The Catlopaedia*. Henston, Guildford.

Evans, J.M. & White, K. (1994) *The Doglopaedia*. Henston, Guildford.

Fox, S. (1988) *Rats*. TFH, USA.

Harkness, J.E. & Wagner, J.E. (1985) *The Biology and Medicine of Rabbits and Rodents.* Lea & Febiger, Philadelphia.

Henwood, C. (1990) *Step by Step – Hamsters.* TFH, USA.

Lane, D. & Cooper, B. (1999) *Veterinary Nursing.* Pergamon Press, Oxford.

McCurnin, D.M. (1994) *Clinical Text for Veterinary Technicians.* W.B. Saunders, Philadelphia.

Morris, D. (1986) *Animal Watching.* Jonathan Cape, London.

Richardson, V.C.G. (1992) *Diseases of Domestic Guinea Pigs.* Blackwell Science, Oxford.

Thies, D. (1989) *Cat Care.* TFH, USA.

## SECTION 3

Bell, C.T.P. (1993) *First Aid and Health Care for Dogs.* Lutterworth Press, Cambridge.

Edney, A.T.B. & Hughes, I.B. (1986) *Pet Care.* Blackwell Science, Oxford.

Fogle, B. (1995) *First Aid for Dogs.* Pelham, London.

Kirk, R.W. & Bistner, S.I. (1985) *Handbook of Veterinary Procedures and Emergency Treatment.* W.B. Saunders, Philadelphia.

Lane, D. & Cooper, B. (1999) *Veterinary Nursing.* Pergamon Press, Oxford.

McBride, D.F. (1996) *Learning Veterinary Terminology.* Mosby, St Louis.

Taylor, D. (1986) *You and Your Cat.* Dorling Kindersley, London.

Taylor, D. (1986) *You and Your Dog.* Dorling Kindersley, London.

# Index